Extranodal Lymphoma from Head to Toe

Editor

MARK D. MURPHEY

RADIOLOGIC CLINICS OF NORTH AMERICA

www.radiologic.theclinics.com

Consulting Editor
FRANK H. MILLER

July 2016 • Volume 54 • Number 4

ELSEVIER

1600 John F. Kennedy Boulevard • Suite 1800 • Philadelphia, Pennsylvania, 19103-2899

http://www.theclinics.com

RADIOLOGIC CLINICS OF NORTH AMERICA Volume 54, Number 4
July 2016 ISSN 0033-8389, ISBN 13: 978-0-323-44855-0

Editor: John Vassallo (j.vassallo@elsevier.com)
Developmental Editor: Donald Mumford

Radiologic Clinics of North America (ISSN 0033-8389) is published bimonthly by Elsevier Inc., 360 Park Avenue South, New York, NY 10010-1710. Months of issue are January, March, May, July, September, and November. Periodicals postage paid at New York, NY and additional mailing offices. Subscription prices are USD 460 per year for US individuals, USD 784 per year for US institutions, USD 100 per year for US students and residents, USD 535 per year for Canadian individuals, USD 1002 per year for Canadian institutions, USD 660 per year for international individuals, USD 1002 per year for international institutions, and USD 315 per year for Canadian and international students/residents. To receive student and resident rate, orders must be accompanied by name of affiliated institution, date of term and the signature of program/residency coordinatior on institution letterhead. Orders will be billed at individual rate until proof of status is received. Foreign air speed delivery is included in all *Clinics* subscription prices. All prices are subject to change without notice. **POSTMASTER:** Send address changes to *Radiologic Clinics of North America*, Elsevier Health Sciences Division, Subscription Customer Service, 3251 Riverport Lane, Maryland Heights, MO63043. **Customer Service: Telephone: 1-800-654-2452** (U.S. and Canada); **1-314-447-8871** (outside U.S. and Canada). **Fax: 1-314-447-8029. E-mail:** journalscustomerservice-usa@elsevier.com **(for print support);** journalsonlinesupport-usa@elsevier.com **(for online support).**

Reprints. For copies of 100 or more of articles in this publication, please contact the Commercial Reprints Department, Elsevier Inc., 360 Park Avenue South, New York, New York 10010-1710. Tel.: +1-212-633-3874; Fax: +1-212-633-3820; E-mail: reprints@elsevier.com.

Radiologic Clinics of North America also published in Greek Paschalidis Medical Publications, Athens, Greece.

Radiologic Clinics of North America is covered in *MEDLINE/PubMed (Index Medicus), EMBASE/Excerpta Medica, Current Contents/Life Sciences, Current Contents/Clinical Medicine, RSNA Index to Imaging Literature, BIOSIS, Science Citation Index,* and *ISI/BIOMED*.

Printed in the United States of America.

Contributors

CONSULTING EDITOR

FRANK H. MILLER, MD
Chief, Body Imaging Section and Fellowship
Program; Medical Director of MRI; Professor,
Department of Radiology, Northwestern
University Feinberg School of Medicine,
Chicago, Illinois

EDITOR

MARK D. MURPHEY, MD, FACR
Physician-in-Chief, International Course
Director, Radiologic Pathology Course
Director, Chief, Musculoskeletal Imaging,
American Institute for Radiologic Pathology,

Professor of Radiology, Uniformed Services
University of the Health Sciences, Staff
Radiologist Musculoskeletal Section, Walter
Reed National Military Medical Center,
Bethesda, Maryland

AUTHORS

AARON AUERBACH, MD, MPH
The Joint Pathology Center, Silver Spring,
Maryland

RAHAT M. BHATTI, MD
Hematopathology Fellow, Department of
Pathology, University of Virginia,
Charlottesville, Virginia

ALLEN P. BURKE, MD
Professor, Department of Pathology, University
of Maryland School of Medicine, Baltimore,
Maryland

ELLEN M. CHUNG, MD, COL, MC, USA
Associate Professor, Vice Chair, Department of
Radiology and Radiological Sciences, F.
Edward Hébert School of Medicine, Uniformed
Services University of the Health Sciences,
Bethesda, Maryland; Chief, Pediatric
Radiology Section, American Institute for
Radiologic Pathology, Silver Spring, Maryland

TERI J. FRANKS, MD
Pulmonary and Mediastinal Pathology,
Department of Defense, Joint Pathology
Center, Silver Spring, Maryland

ALETTA ANN FRAZIER, MD
Associate Professor, Department of
Diagnostic Radiology and Nuclear Medicine,
University of Maryland School of Medicine,
Baltimore, Maryland; American Institute for
Radiologic Pathology, Silver Spring,
Maryland

JEFFREY R. GALVIN, MD
Chest Imaging, Department of Radiology
and Nuclear Medicine and Pulmonary and
Critical Care Medicine, Department of
Internal Medicine, University of Maryland
School of Medicine, Baltimore, Maryland;
Chest Imaging, American Institute for
Radiologic Pathology, Silver Spring,
Maryland

LEONARD GLASSMAN, MD
Washington Radiology Associates PC,
Washington, DC

EMILY HECKENDORN, DO
Walter Reed National Medical Military Center,
Bethesda, Maryland

JEAN JEUDY, MD
Associate Professor, Department of Diagnostic
Radiology and Nuclear Medicine, University of
Maryland School of Medicine, Baltimore,
Maryland

SETH J. KLIGERMAN, MD
Chest Imaging, Department of Radiology and
Nuclear Medicine, University of Maryland
School of Medicine, Baltimore, Maryland;
Chest Imaging, American Institute for
Radiologic Pathology, Silver Spring, Maryland

KELLY K. KOELLER, MD, FACR
Associate Professor, Department of Radiology,
Mayo Clinic, Rochester, Minnesota; American
Institute for Radiologic Pathology,
Neuroradiology Section, Silver Spring,
Maryland

MARK J. KRANSDORF, MD
Department of Radiology, Mayo Clinic
Hospital, Phoenix, Arizona

GRANT E. LATTIN Jr, MD, Lt Col, USAF, MC
Department of Radiology and Radiological
Sciences, F. Edward Hébert School of
Medicine, Uniformed Services University of the
Health Sciences, Bethesda, Maryland;
American Institute for Radiologic Pathology,
Silver Spring, Maryland

MARC S. LEVINE, MD
Department of Radiology, Hospital of the
University of Pennsylvania, Philadelphia,
Pennsylvania

MARIA A. MANNING, MD
Gastrointestinal Section Chief, American
Institute for Radiologic Pathology, Silver
Spring, Maryland; Associate Professor,
Division of Abdominal Imaging, Department of
Radiology, MedStar Georgetown University
Hospital, Washington, DC

ANUPAMJIT K. MEHROTRA, MD
The Joint Pathology Center, Silver Spring,
Maryland

MARK D. MURPHEY, MD, FACR
Physician-in-Chief, International Course
Director, Radiologic Pathology Course

Director, Chief, Musculoskeletal Imaging,
American Institute for Radiologic Pathology,
Professor of Radiology, Uniformed Services
University of the Health Sciences, Staff
Radiologist Musculoskeletal Section, Walter
Reed National Military Medical Center,
Bethesda, Maryland

BRANDI T. NICHOLSON, MD
Associate Professor of Radiology, Department
of Radiology and Medical Imaging, University
of Virginia, Charlottesville, Virginia

MICHAEL PAVIO, BS, 2LT, MSC, USA
Fourth-year Medical Student, F. Edward
Hébert School of Medicine, Uniformed
Services University of the Health Sciences,
Bethesda, Maryland

**IVÁN R. ROHENA-QUINQUILLA, MD, MAJ,
USA, MC**
Department of Radiology and Radiological
Sciences, F. Edward Hébert School of
Medicine, Uniformed Services University of the
Health Sciences, Bethesda, Maryland;
Department of Radiology, Martin Army
Community Hospital, Fort Benning, Georgia

ROBERT Y. SHIH, LTC, MC, USA
Assistant Professor, Department of Radiology,
Walter Reed National Military Medical Center,
Uniformed Services University of the Health
Sciences, Bethesda, Maryland; American
Institute for Radiologic Pathology,
Neuroradiology Section, Silver Spring,
Maryland

ALEXANDER S. SOMWARU, MD
Division of Abdominal Imaging, Department of
Radiology, MedStar Georgetown University
Hospital, Washington, DC

DARCY WOLFMAN, MD
Department of Radiology and Radiological
Sciences, F. Edward Hébert School of
Medicine, Uniformed Services University of the
Health Sciences; Department of Radiology,
Walter Reed National Military Medical Center,
Bethesda, Maryland; Section Chief of
Genitourinary Imaging, American Institute for
Radiologic Pathology, Silver Spring, Maryland

Contents

of epicardium and pericardium. Pericardial implants and effusions are common. The disease is often multifocal in the heart, but cardiac valves are usually spared.

Primary lymphoma of bone and soft tissue is rare and almost invariably of B-cell origin. Osseous lymphoma usually reveals aggressive bone destruction and associated soft tissue extension. Soft tissue involvement is optimally depicted by MR imaging. Cortical destruction allowing communication between the intraosseous and soft tissue components may be subtle with small striations of extension. Lymphoma of the deep soft tissues usually reveals long cones of intramuscular or intermuscular tumor again best depicted by MR imaging. Cutaneous or subcutaneous lymphoma demonstrates multiple nodules and plaquelike thickening.

PROGRAM OBJECTIVE

The objective of the *Radiologic Clinics of North America* is to keep practicing radiologists and radiology residents up to date with current clinical practice in radiology by providing timely articles reviewing the state of the art in patient care.

TARGET AUDIENCE

Practicing radiologists, radiology residents, and other health care professionals who provide patient care utilizing radiologic findings.

LEARNING OBJECTIVES

Upon completion of this activity, participants will be able to:
1. Review the pathology of extranodal lymphoma.
2. Discuss the presentation of extranodal lymphoma in various body systems such as the gastrointestinal, cardiothoracic, and genitourinary systems.
3. Recognize imaging methods in pediatric extranodal lymphoma.

ACCREDITATION

The Elsevier Office of Continuing Medical Education (EOCME) is accredited by the Accreditation Council for Continuing Medical Education (ACCME) to provide continuing medical education for physicians.

The EOCME designates this enduring material for a maximum of 15 *AMA PRA Category 1 Credit*(s)™. Physicians should claim only the credit commensurate with the extent of their participation in the activity.

All other health care professionals requesting continuing education credit for this enduring material will be issued a certificate of participation.

DISCLOSURE OF CONFLICTS OF INTEREST

The EOCME assesses conflict of interest with its instructors, faculty, planners, and other individuals who are in a position to control the content of CME activities. All relevant conflicts of interest that are identified are thoroughly vetted by EOCME for fair balance, scientific objectivity, and patient care recommendations. EOCME is committed to providing its learners with CME activities that promote improvements or quality in healthcare and not a specific proprietary business or a commercial interest.

The planning committee, staff, authors and editors listed below have identified no financial relationships or relationships to products or devices they or their spouse/life partner have with commercial interest related to the content of this CME activity:

Aaron Auerbach, MD, MPH; Rahat M. Bhatti, MD; Allen P. Burke, MD; Ellen M. Chung, MD, COL, MC, USA; Anjali Fortna; Teri J. Franks, MD; Aletta Ann Frazier, MD; Jeffrey R. Galvin, MD; Leonard Glassman, MD; Emily Heckendorn, DO; Jean Jeudy, MD; Seth J. Kligerman, MD; Kelly K. Koeller, MD, FACR; Mark J. Kransdorf, MD; Grant E. Lattin Jr, MD, Lt Col, USAF, MC; Maria A. Manning, MD; Anupamjit K. Mehrotra, MD; Mark D. Murphey, MD, FACR; Brandi T. Nicholson, MD; Michael Pavio, BS, 2LT, MSC, USA; Iván R. Rohena-Quinquilla, MD, MAJ, USA, MC; Erin Scheckenbach; Robert Y. Shih, LTC, MC, USA; Alexander S. Somwaru, MD; Karthik Subramaniam; John Vassallo; Darcy Wolfman, MD.

The planning committee, staff, authors and editors listed below have identified financial relationships or relationships to products or devices they or their spouse/life partner have with commercial interest related to the content of this CME activity:

Marc S. Levine, MD is a consultant/advisor for Bracco Diagnostic Inc., and receives royalties/patents from Elsevier B.V. and Cambridge University Press.

UNAPPROVED/OFF-LABEL USE DISCLOSURE

The EOCME requires CME faculty to disclose to the participants:
1. When products or procedures being discussed are off-label, unlabelled, experimental, and/or investigational (not US Food and Drug Administration [FDA] approved); and
2. Any limitations on the information presented, such as data that are preliminary or that represent ongoing research, interim analyses, and/or unsupported opinions. Faculty may discuss information about pharmaceutical agents that is outside of FDA-approved labelling. This information is intended solely for CME and is not intended to promote off-label use of these medications. If you have any questions, contact the medical affairs department of the manufacturer for the most recent prescribing information.

TO ENROLL

To enroll in the *Radiologic Clinics of North America* Continuing Medical Education program, call customer service at 1-800-654-2452 or sign up online at http://www.theclinics.com/home/cme. The CME program is available to subscribers for an additional annual fee of USD 315.

METHOD OF PARTICIPATION

In order to claim credit, participants must complete the following:

1. Complete enrolment as indicated above.
2. Read the activity.
3. Complete the CME Test and Evaluation. Participants must achieve a score of 70% on the test. All CME Tests and Evaluations must be completed online.

CME INQUIRIES/SPECIAL NEEDS

For all CME inquiries or special needs, please contact elsevierCME@elsevier.com.

RADIOLOGIC CLINICS OF NORTH AMERICA

THE CLINICS ARE AVAILABLE ONLINE!
Access your subscription at:
www.theclinics.com

Preface
Imaging of Extranodal Lymphoma

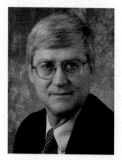

Mark D. Murphey, MD, FACR
Editor

Lymphoid neoplasms represent a common group of malignancies that confront radiologists on a daily basis. In fact, it is estimated that lymphoma will become the most frequent cancer within the next 20 years. This marked increase in incidence of lymphoma is being caused by both the aging population of many cultures and the dramatic rise in the number of immunocompromised patients. Radiologists of all subspecialties need to be aware of this increasing disease prevalence of lymphoma in our society and its myriad of imaging appearances. The imaging characteristics of lymphoma are often characteristic or suggestive of the diagnosis throughout the various organ systems that are affected.

Cross-sectional imaging, including ultrasonography, CT, and MR imaging, is vital in the detection, characterization, and staging of lymphomatous masses throughout the body. FDG-PET imaging has revolutionized our ability to identify areas of systemic lymphomatous involvement because of the intense radionuclide avidity seen. These imaging modalities have also allowed radiologists to be at the forefront in continued assessment of patients to evaluate therapeutic effects of treatment and evaluate for recurrence of lymphomatous involvement.

The classification of lymphoma is a continuing dynamic process that is constantly changing. In this issue of *Radiologic Clinics of North America*, my colleagues at the American Institute for Radiologic Pathology (AIRP) have provided an extensive update of the radiologic and pathologic assessment of extranodal lymphoma from head to toe. Our emphasis at the AIRP is the importance of radiologic–pathologic correlation in imaging diagnosis and assessment, which is illustrated in this issue on extranodal lymphoma. Understanding that the radiologic appearance is a direct reflection of the pathologic process is vital to improving our diagnostic acumen and facilitating our patients' management, care, and outcome. It is hoped that this issue provides a useful review and resource of the radiologic and pathologic assessment of extranodal lymphoma and helps guide our evaluation from diagnosis and throughout the disease course.

Mark D. Murphey, MD, FACR
Physician-in-chief
Chief, Musculoskeletal Imaging
American Institute for Radiologic Pathology
Uniformed Services University of the Health
Sciences
Walter Reed National Military Medical Center
Bethesda, MD 20889, USA

E-mail address:
mmurphey@acr.org

Radiol Clin N Am 54 (2016) xi
http://dx.doi.org/10.1016/j.rcl.2016.04.002
0033-8389/16/$ – see front matter © 2016 Elsevier Inc. All rights reserved.

Pathology of Extranodal Lymphoma

Emily Heckendorn, DO[a], Aaron Auerbach, MD, MPH[b],*

KEYWORDS

• Extranodal lymphoma • Classification • Immunohistochemistry • Molecular oncology

KEY POINTS

• The 2008 *WHO Classification of Tumours of Haematopoietic and Lymphoid Tissues* is the current international gold standard for identifying and classifying tumors of hematopoietic and lymphoid origin.
• Phenotyping by immunohistochemistry (IHC) and flow cytometry as well as determining lymphoma-specific molecular alterations are essential parts of the criteria for diagnosing different types of extranodal lymphomas.
• B-cell neoplasms are generally divided into 3 categories: B-lymphoblastic leukemia/lymphoma (precursor B-lymphoid neoplasms), mature B-cell neoplasms, and Hodgkin lymphoma.
• The gastrointestinal (GI) tract is the most common site of extranodal lymphomas, and marginal zone lymphoma is the most common extranodal B-cell lymphoma.
• Different types of T-cell lymphomas are seen predominantly in certain specific extranodal locations, that is, enteropathy-associated T-cell lymphoma (EATL) is usually seen in the GI tract and hepatosplenic T-cell lymphoma is typically seen in the bone marrow, spleen, and liver.

INTRODUCTION TO CLASSIFICATION

The realm of lymphoma classification is dynamic and constantly changing. The 2008 *WHO Classification of Tumours* is the current international gold standard for identifying and classifying tumors of hematopathic and lymphoid origin. The strength of this text is that it organizes different lymphomas into distinct tumors that have discrete diagnostic criteria. Lymphoid neoplasms comprise the sixth most common group of malignancies worldwide and are predicted to become the most common form of cancer within the next 20 years.[1] We are on the eve of revising the 2008 World Health Organization (WHO) text. With advances in molecular oncology as well as insights into phenotyping by Immunohistochemistry (IHC) and flow cytometry, lymphomas are being reclassified to reflect changes in prognosis and changes in treatment.

There are 2 main types of lymphoma: B-cell lymphoma and T-cell lymphoma, with B-cell lymphomas vastly outnumbering T-cell lymphomas. B-cell neoplasms are generally divided into 3 categories: B-lymphoblastic leukemia/lymphoma (precursor B-lymphoid neoplasms), mature B-cell neoplasms, and Hodgkin lymphoma. Mature B-cell lymphomas may be further classified based on size into small B-cell lymphomas and large (high-grade) B-cell lymphomas. The 2008 WHO classification includes 22 different types of T-cell and natural killer (NK)-cell lymphomas, grouped into leukemic, extranodal, nodal, and cutaneous.[2] Precursor B-cell and T-cell lymphomas occur primarily in the lymph nodes and bone marrow, and T-lymphoblastic leukemia/T-lymphoblastic lymphoma (T-LBL) commonly involves the mediastinum.

Disclosure: The opinions and assertions herein are the private views of the authors and are not to be construed as official or as reflecting the views of the Department of the Army or the Department of Defense.
[a] Walter Reed National Medical Military Center, Bethesda, MD, USA; [b] The Joint Pathology Center, Silver Spring, MD, USA
* Corresponding author.
E-mail address: Aaron.auerbach.civ@mail.mil

Radiol Clin N Am 54 (2016) 639–648
http://dx.doi.org/10.1016/j.rcl.2016.03.001
0033-8389/16/$ – see front matter Published by Elsevier Inc.

A patient's clinical history along with a variety of laboratory methods is of critical importance to correctly identify most types of lymphoma. In the laboratory, a combination of morphology, IHC for phenotyping, and flow cytometry for phenotyping and molecular testing is used to accurately classify a lymphoma. Tumor morphology is viewed through a process of formalin fixation, chemical processing, sectioning, and staining of tissue and allows pathologists to examine the architecture, cytology, and overall morphology of the specimen. Hematoxylin-eosin (H&E) is the characteristic stain used. Traditionally, IHC and molecular studies have been used as adjuncts to the morphology to confirm a diagnosis; however, with increasing frequency, IHC and molecular tests are essential to classifying lymphomas that appear morphologically identical on H&E but have substantial clinical implications in regard to prognosis or treatment. By immunophenotyping and molecular analysis, specific antigens and genes are identified that can serve as prognostic markers and may allow for potential treatment targets.

IMMUNOPHENOTYPING

Although lymphocytes can be morphologically similar, they are extremely heterogeneous in lineage, function, and phenotype.[3] Cells are distinguished by surface proteins through panels of monoclonal antibodies, a process called IHC staining. The standard nomenclature for many of these antigens is cluster of differentiation (CD). CDs are used to delineate surface proteins that define a particular cell type or stage of differentiation.[3] To demonstrate a neoplastic process, proof of monoclonality is typically needed. Monoclonality of a B-cell proliferation can be identified based on kappa and lambda staining. Normally kappa and lambda are expressed in a 3:1 ratio. A predominance of kappa light chain B cells or lambda light chain B cells indicates monoclonality,

generally implying a neoplastic proliferation.[4] Furthermore, a mixed population of kappa and lambda B cells favors a reactive process. When classifying a lymphoma, the specific cell lineage, B cell or T cell, must be identified. This is usually determined by performing a series of IHC panels identifying specific B-cell or T-cell markers. Mature B-cell markers include CD19, CD20, and CD79a. CD2, CD3, CD5, CD7, and CD43 are considered T-cell markers. T-cell lymphomas, however, also frequently show loss of 1 or more of these T-cell markers, so multiple markers are needed for diagnosis of a T-cell neoplasm (**Fig. 1**). For example, CD7 is the most common T-cell marker lost in the T-cell lymphoma, mycosis fungoides.

Some IHC markers indicate parts of a reactive lymph node. Markers, such as GCET1, CD10, and BCL-6, highlight B cells of the germinal center, whereas PD1 and CXCL13 mark T cells in the germinal center (follicular helper T cells). IgD selectively marks the mantle zone of a lymph node. Furthermore, specific lymphomas are derived from these lymph node compartments. For example, follicular lymphoma originates from germinal center B cells and expresses GCET1, CD10, and BCL6[+], whereas angioimmunoblastic lymphoma is derived from germinal center T cells and expresses PD1 and CXCL13.[5]

GENETIC TESTING

Molecular testing is an important adjunct to the histologic examination of lymphomas. Polymerase chain reaction (PCR), fluorescence in situ hybridization (FISH), cytogenetics, and next-generation sequencing studies are all used to make the diagnosis of lymphoma. B-cell and T-cell proliferations can be evaluated for monoclonality by the presence of immunoglobulin or T-cell receptor rearrangements, which are typically performed by PCR (**Fig. 2**). Molecular testing for specific

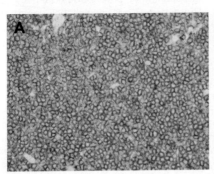

Fig. 1. Use of T-cell IHC in mature T-cell lymphomas. (*A*) CD3 is strongly positive in this case of EATL (CD3 immunohistochemical stain, original magnification, 10×). (*B*) The lymphoyctes are negative in the same case. Loss of T-cell markers, such as CD2 in this case, is a feature of T-cell lymphoma (CD2 immunohistochemical stain, original magnification, 20×).

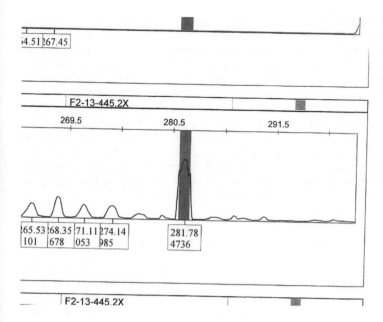

Fig. 2. Monoclonality for *IGH* gene rearrangement in B-cell lymphoma. This is an image of a PCR test for *IGH* gene rearrangement. The pink band represents a dominant monoclonal peak for *IGH* at position 281. *IGH* monoclonality is a feature of B-cell lymphoma.

translocations and specific gene mutations can be performed by FISH or cytogenetics.

Being able to recognize extranodal lymphomas is of utmost importance. Although lymphomas originating in lymph nodes are more common, extranodal lymphomas are generally considered more difficult to diagnose than nodal-based lymphomas. This is in part because there are reactive inflammatory processes in extranodal sites, which are in the differential diagnosis. For example, *Helicobacter pylori* (H pylori) infection presents with a gastric lymphoid infiltrate that may look similar to gastric marginal zone lymphoma, particularly on a small core needle biopsy. Extranodal lymphomas are often misdiagnosed as reactive hyperplasia, or pseudolymphomas, and are a frequent cause of medical malpractice for pathologists.

Extranodal lymphomas also seem to be increasing in frequency. This may be attributed to the increase in recognition of marginal zone B-cell lymphomas that were previously diagnosed as hyperplasia or pseudolymphoma. The most common sites of extranodal lymphoma in order, of decreasing frequently, include stomach, skin, oral cavity/pharynx, small intestine, brain, colon/rectum, thyroid, soft tissue, lung/pleura, and orbit.

LYMPHOMAS INVOLVING THE GASTROINTESTINAL TRACT

The GI tract is the most common site of extranodal lymphomas; 20% to 25% of primary extranodal lymphomas occur in the GI tract.[6] However, primary GI lymphomas account for only 1% to 4% of all GI tumors.[7] A large variety of lymphoma types may develop as primary intestinal neoplasms. A few entities, such as EATL, are unique to the GI system; many others, such as diffuse large B-cell lymphoma (DLBCL), marginal zone lymphoma, and chronic lymphocytic lymphoma, are also commonly found outside the GI system.[8] The intestines may also be a presenting site of secondary involvement of lymphoma.[6] Risk factors of GI lymphomas include infection with H pylori for marginal zone lymphoma, Epstein-Barr virus (EBV) for Burkitt lymphoma (BL), celiac disease for EATL, and immune deficiency.

The stomach is the most frequent site of GI involvement by lymphoma, most commonly by marginal zone lymphoma.[8] The differential diagnosis of GI involvement by small lymphocytes is long but includes reactive follicular hyperplasia, H pylori gastritis, marginal zone lymphoma, mantle cell lymphoma, follicular lymphoma, and small lymphocytic lymphoma.[7]

Extranodal Marginal Zone Lymphoma

First described by Issacson and Wright in 1983, extranodal marginal zone lymphoma is a B-cell lymphoma composed of small monomorphic cells, which is often associated with an autoimmune disease or infectious disease process. Extranodal marginal zone lymphoma can occur at multiple anatomic sites, the most common being the stomach,[7] where it is thought to evolve from native mucosa-associated lymphoid tissue (MALT). Extranodal marginal zone lymphoma is associated with infectious organisms, such as *H pylori* in the stomach, *Campylobacter jejuni* in the small intestine, *Chlamydia psittaci* in the ocular region, and *Borrelia burgdorferi* in the skin.[9] Associated autoimmune diseases include Hashimoto thyroiditis in the thyroid and Sjögren syndrome in the salivary glands.[9]

The differential diagnosis includes reactive inflammatory processes. Malignant features of extranodal marginal zone lymphoma that distinguish it from a reactive process include colonization of germinal centers, monocytoid appearance, plasmacytoid cells with Dutcher bodies, confluence of marginal zones, and lymphoepithelial lesions[8] (Fig. 3). The neoplastic cells infiltrate around reactive germinal centers and eventually overrun the follicles. Frequently, the malignant cells have pale-staining cytoplasm, giving the appearance of a monocyte. Plasmacytic differentiation is present in approximately one-third of cases.[9] Lymphoepithelial lesions are aggregates of neoplastic lesions with distortion or destruction of the epithelium.

There is no specific antigenic marker for extranodal marginal zone lymphomas; however, a panel of immunostains is used to eliminate other lymphomas. Similar to almost all mature B-cell neoplasms, extranodal marginal zone lymphomas are positive for CD20, BCL-2, and CD43. BCL-6, cyclin D1, and CD10 are negative. CD5 is usually negative but may on occasion be positive.[9] CD21 and CD23 mark expanded dendritic meshworks in the reactive germinal centers of marginal zone lymphoma, which help distinguish it from reactive follicular hyperplasia or other small B-cell lymphomas.

Extranodal marginal zone lymphoma is associated with multiple translocations. Each translocation is found with varying frequency corresponding to the site of lymphoma involvement. T(11;18) is associated with stomach and lung sites of involvement and is a unique marker for resistance to *H pylori* antibiotic treatment[7] (Fig. 4). Other translocations are as follows: t(14:18) in salivary glands and eye, t(3;18) in the eye and thyroid, and t(1;14) in intestines and lung.[9] There are multiple areas of overlap, however, between each anatomic site and the translocation involved. In addition to various translocations, trisomies of 3 and 18 are frequently identified. Although this is an indolent tumor, it may transform to DLBCL.[9]

Burkitt Lymphoma

Like marginal zone lymphoma, BL is a B-cell lymphoma that is often extranodal and commonly involves the GI tract. BL commonly affects children and young adults. Three clinical variants are recognized: endemic, sporadic, and immunodeficiency associated. In all 3 clinical variants, patients are at risk for central nervous system (CNS) involvement.[9] In endemic BL, the jaws and other facial bones are the most common site of involvement; however, the GI tract, thyroid, salivary glands, and breasts may also be affected. In a majority of sporadic BLs, the abdomen is the primary site of involvement.[9] Immunodeficiency-associated BL frequently affects lymph nodes and bone marrow.

Unlike marginal zone lymphoma, which is made of small B cells, BL is made of large B cells. The B cells are of germinal center type, so they express CD10 and BCL6. Characteristically, BL has an extremely high proliferation rate and *MYC* translocations (detected by FISH and cytogenetics), although this is not a specific feature. The 3 variants have differing rates of association with EBV, with

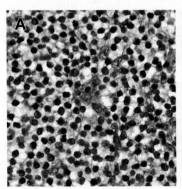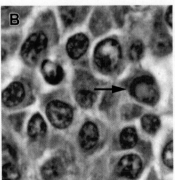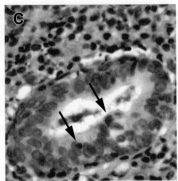

Fig. 3. Morphologic features of marginal zone lymphoma. (*A*) Marginal zone lymphoma can have a monocytoid appearance. The cells have increased clear cytoplasm (Hemotoxylin-eosin stain, original magnification, 20×). (*B*) Dutcher bodies are another feature of marginal zone lymphoma, seen here as a pink intranuclear inclusion (Hemotoxylin-eosin stain, original magnification, 100×). (*C*) Lymphoepithelial lesions are seen in marginal zone lymphoma. This gland has lymphocytes penetrating it (Hemotoxylin-eosin stain, original magnification, 40×).

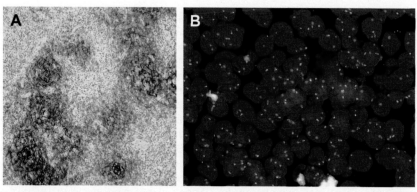

Fig. 4. (*A*) This is an IHC stain for CD21 that shows a disrupted follicular dendritic meshwork, which is a classic feature of marginal zone lymphoma (CD21 immunohistochemical stain, original magnification, 10×). (*B*) *BIRC3/MALT1* t(11;18)(q21;q21) FISH assay. Marginal zone lymphoma, from extra-nodal locations frequently show *BIRC3/MALT1*. The yellow signals indicates the translocation of the *BIRC3 and MALT1* genes (original magnification, 60×).

EBV present in a majority of endemic cases and detected in approximately 30% of sporadic and 25% to 40% of immunodeficiency-associated cases.[9] BL has the highest Ki-67 expression of any lymphoma, with a nearly 100% proliferation rate. This high proliferation index gives BL the characteristic histologic appearance of a starry sky, which is caused by the numerous benign macrophages ingesting apoptotic debris (**Fig. 5**). DLBCL is within the differential diagnosis of BL but typically does not show a proliferation rate of greater than 90%. BCL2 is either negative or weakly positive in BL, which can differentiate it from DLBCL, which may show strong BCL2 positivity.

Follicular Lymphoma

Most primary follicular lymphomas in the GI tract are located in the small intestine, specifically in the second portion of the duodenum. This lymphoma may be an incidental finding during endoscopy and may present as multiple small polyps. Patients with duodenal follicular lymphoma typically have low-stage localized disease and have a favorable prognosis, even if the lymphoma is not treated. The morphology and phenotype of duodenal follicular lymphoma is similar to follicular lymphoma elsewhere and is composed of germinal center B cells, staining positive for CD10, BCL-6, and other B-cell markers (CD20 and CD79a).[9]

Mantle Cell Lymphoma

Mantle cell lymphoma is an aggressive lymphoma and when it presents extranodally, it is commonly found in the terminal ileum and ileocecal valve.[7] The term, *lymphomatoid papulosis*, is given to cases of mantle cell lymphomas that stud along the GI tract. Mantle cell lymphoma expresses B-cell markers, CD5, CD43, and BCL-2, as well as cell-cycle markers, cyclin D1 and SOX11.[7]

PRIMARY CUTANEOUS LYMPHOMAS

Primary cutaneous lymphomas are the second most common site of extranodal lymphomas. By

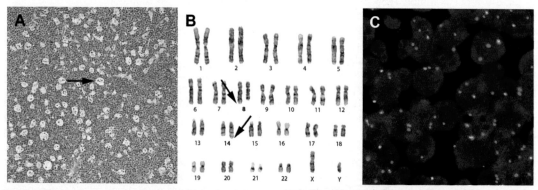

Fig. 5. (*A*) BL shows sheets of intermediate-sized B-cells with evenly interspersed reactive, tingible body macrophages imparting a characteristic starry sky pattern (Hemotoxylin-eosin stain, original magnification, 20×). (*B*) Cytogenetic karyotype. A t(8;14) (q24;32) involving a *MYC* gene rearrangement is identified in this karyotype of a patient with BL. This is the most common translocation of BL. (*C*) *MYC* gene FISH break apart study. *MYC* rearrangement is identified by seeing 1 red, 1 green, and 1 yellow signal in each cell (original magnification, 100×).

definition, these are limited to cases that manifest exclusively in the skin with no extracutaneous disease at diagnosis or within 6 months. The most common types of cutaneous lymphoma include mycosis fungoides and primary cutaneous anaplastic large cell lymphoma. Mycosis fungoides characteristically shows epidermotropism and a slowly evolving patch to plaque to tumor progression. Primary cutaneous anaplastic large cell lymphoma is notable for a dermal CD30[+] infiltrate and is classified separately from ALK[+] anaplastic large cell lymphoma. Primary cutaneous anaplastic large cell lymphoma is distinct in that it is ALK and EMA negative. Furthermore, the IRF4/MUM1 oncogene on chromosome 6p25.3 is mutated in approximately 30% of primary cutaneous anaplastic large cell lymphoma cases but only rarely in systemic anaplastic large cell lymphoma. Expression of IRF4/MUM1 protein by IHC does not correlate with the presence of the translocation and cannot be used as a surrogate marker. Newer skin lymphomas that are provisional diagnoses in the 2008 WHO classification include primary cutaneous CD4[+] small medium T-cell lymphoma and primary cutaneous CD8[+] aggressive epidermotropic cytotoxic T-cell lymphoma.

SOFT TISSUE

Soft tissue involvement by lymphoma usually represents either a systemic lymphoma that has soft tissue involvement or contiguous involvement of the soft tissue of a lymphoma that is involving a lymph node. Lymphomas primary to the soft tissue are exceedingly uncommon, representing approximately 1% of the soft tissue tumors of a consultation practice.[10] DLBCL is the most commonly occurring lymphoma in the United States[11] and is by far the most common type of lymphoma to involve the soft tissue. In 1 study, DLBCL comprised 57% of lymphomas in the soft tissue.[12] DLBCL can occur as a primary entity or transform from a previous malignancy (follicular lymphoma, marginal zone lymphoma, chronic lymphocytic leukemia/small cell lymphocytic lymphoma, or nodular lymphocyte-predominant Hodgkin lymphoma [NLPHL]).[9] Immunodeficiency is a significant risk factor.

Besides the GI tract and soft tissue, DLBCL may also occur in lymph nodes as well as bone, testis, spleen, thyroid, and kidney. DLBCLs most commonly occur in the elderly (median age is in the 7th decade), although children can be affected.[9] Most patients are asymptomatic; when symptoms are present, they are generally dependent on the site of tumor involvement.

The WHO defines DLBCL as a neoplasm with nuclei more than twice the size of a normal lymphocyte that has a diffuse growth pattern. Clinical, immunotypical, and molecular features have subdivided DLBCL into distinct disease entities. DLBCL remains a heterogeneous category of tumors, with cell-of-origin studies revealing 2 distinct subtypes: activated B-cell (ABC) and germinal center B-cell (GCB) types. GCB type DLBCL is associated with a better prognosis in comparison to the ABC type. Testing of GCB versus ABC type can be performed by IHC or gene expression profiling, with the latter the more preferred method.[13] Several systems exist for IHC identification of GCB type; one of the best known is the Hans classifier, which identifies the GCB type as either a DLBCL that is CD10[+] or CD10[−], BCL6[+], and MUM1[−].[13] CD10 and BCL6 are normally positive in germinal centers, and MUM1 is mutually exclusive with BCL6.

Morphologically, DLBCL has a diffuse to vaguely nodular pattern of involvement. Pan B-cell markers are expressed: CD19, CD20, CD22, and CD79a[9]; 1 one or more may be lacking. BCL2 expression is an adverse prognostic marker, associated with the ABC type. BCL2 expression is not necessarily related to the presence or absence of t(14;18).[13] Although classically associated with BL, MYC rearrangement is seen in 6% to 16% of cases of DLBCL.[11] Given the relative frequency of DLBCL compared with BL, there are more MYC-positive DLBCL cases than BL cases.[11] IHC can now be used to detect MYC protein expression, although it is not yet widely used.[11] A double-hit lymphoma is defined as a MYC abnormality with another genetic abnormality,[11] such as BCL2 or BCL6 mutations. BCL-2 rearrangements with a MYC breakpoint is the most common double-hit mutation. These cases have a significantly worse prognosis than just 1 adverse prognostic marker.[11]

Lymphomas Involving the Mediastinum

Primary mediastinal B-cell lymphoma

Primary mediastinal B-cell lymphoma (PMBL) is a diffuse medium to large B-cell lymphoma primarily occurring in young female adults. Presenting symptoms are frequently related to the large size of the tumor; patients may present with superior vena cava syndrome. The lymphoma is characterized by large cells with abundant clear cytoplasm and compartmentalizing fibrosis; however, these characteristics are not always present and there are no pathognomonic morphologic features to distinguish PMBL from DLBCL.[14] Genetic analysis reveals gains in segments of chromosome 9 in approximately 50% of PMBL.[14] Gains in segments of chromosome 2 and X can also be present.[9,14] PMBL has variable expression of BCL-6 and BCL-2.[9] CD30 is positive in a majority of cases but is usually weak and heterogeneous, unlike Hodgkin lymphoma.[9] Unlike DLBC, PMBL frequently overexpresses and stains MAL and TRAF. Overexpression of the *MAL* gene is the most specific oncogene abnormality in PMBL.[14]

Hodgkin lymphoma

Hodgkin lymphoma frequently involves the mediastinum, and it is nodular sclerosis classical Hodgkin lymphoma (CHL) that is mostly mediastinal. Hodgkin lymphoma is a unique category of B-cell lymphoma with distinct morphologic and IHC features. Hodgkin is divided into 2 diseases entities: NLPHL and CHL. NLPHL is characterized by the lymphocyte-predominant cell, formerly known as a popcorn cell, a large, neoplastic cell with a large folded nucleus. Lymphocyte-predominant cells are positive for PAX5, CD10, CD20, CD79a, and CD45 and lack expression of CD15 and CD30, unlike CHL. NLPHL is not associated with EBV. The main mimicker of NLPHL is T-cell–rich B-cell lymphoma (TCRBCL): both have large, malignant, CD20$^+$ cells in a background of benign T cells. NLPHL can be distinguished from TCRBCL by the preservation of the CD21$^+$ and CD23$^+$ follicular dendritic network and the presence of CD4$^+$ T cells. TCRBCL lacks a follicular dendritic network and has CD8$^+$ T cells.

The characteristic Reed-Sternberg cell of CHL has at least 2 nucleoli in 2 separate nuclear lobes. Mononuclear variants are termed, *Hodgkin cells*. Both Reed-Sternberg and Hodgkin cells are positive for CD30 in nearly all cases and CD15 in a lesser extent. B-cell markers, CD20, PAX5, and

MUM1, may be detectable but are usually weakly staining[9] (**Fig. 6**). CD79a is rarely expressed. CHL is divided into 4 entities: nodular CHL (NSCHL), mixed cellularity CHL (MCCHL), lymphocyte-rich CHL, and lymphocyte-depleted CHL. EBV can be found in all cases of CHL but is found primarily in MCCHL and lymphocyte-depleted CHL.

NSCHL involves the mediastinum in 80% of cases and accounts for approximately 70% of CHLs in Europe and the United States.[9] NSCHL has a variant of the Reed-Sternberg cell, termed, *the lacunar cell*, which shows retraction artifact of the cytoplasm so that the cells seem to be in lacunae. Collagenous sclerosis surrounds nodules and is usually associated with a thickened lymph node capsule. A mixed inflammatory infiltrate of eosinophils, histiocytes, and neutrophils is often present. NSCHL has the best prognosis of all the CHL.

MCCHL is more frequent in HIV patients. Mediastinal involvement is uncommon. MCCHL lacks fibrosis and EBER is expressed in approximately 75% of cases.[9] Lymphocyte-rich CHL has a nodular growth pattern that may have small or regressed germinal centers. The Reed-Sternberg and Hodgkin cells are found in the mantle zone. Neutrophils and eosinophils are absent. Morphologically, this subtype can be confused with NLPHL, but IHC stains distinguish the two. Lymphocyte-depleted CHL has a relative predominance of Hodgkin and Reed-Sternberg cells in comparison with the background lymphocytes. This subtype is the rarest CHL and is often associated with HIV.

T-lymphoblastic lymphoma

T-LBL is a precursor T-cell neoplasm that frequently involves the mediastinum. It may also

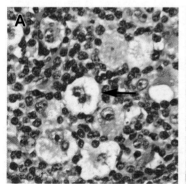 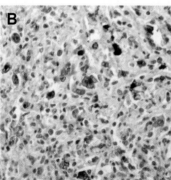 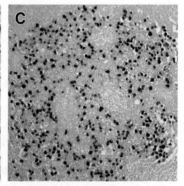

Fig. 6. (*A*) There are scattered Reed-Sternberg cells, which are large cells, some binucleate, with prominent nucleoli sitting within lacunar spaces (Hemotoxylin-eosin stain, original magnification, 40×). (*B*) There are scattered CD30 positive Reed-Sternberg cells showing a mem-branous and Golgi pattern of staining (CD30 immunohistochemical stain, original magnification, 20×). (*C*) EBER in situ hybridication test. EBER is positive in the Reed-Sternberg cells of a case of CHL. EBER is positive in approximately 50% of cases of CHL (original magnification, 10×).

involve the tonsils, liver, spleen, CNS, testis, and skin.[9] The neoplastic cells look immature and may phenotypically be CD4 and CD8 double positive or double negative. The most specific markers to indicate the precursor nature of T lymphoblasts are Tdt, CD34, CD1a, and CD99. The primary histologic mimicker of T-LBL is a thymoma. Thymomas, unlike T-LBL, contain epithelioid cells that stain for cytokeratins, p63, and PAX8.

B-cell Lymphomas in the Lungs and Pleural Cavity

Primary lung lymphomas are a rare entity, accounting for 0.4% of all lymphomas.[15] The most common primary lung lymphoma is marginal zone lymphoma (discussed previously).

Lymphomatoid granulomatosis
Lymphomatoid granulomatosis is an EBV-driven, angiocentric, and angiodestructive lymphoproliferative disease involving the lungs in more than 90% of cases.[9] Other common sites of involvement include the brain, kidney, liver, and skin.[9] It is a rare disease primarily affecting immunodeficient adults. It most commonly presents as bilateral pulmonary nodules that vary in size.[16] The malignant cells are positive for B-cell markers by IHC and EBER with in situ hybridization. Cases are graded based on the number of EBV-positive cells and the prognosis is poor.

Primary effusion lymphoma
Primary effusion lymphoma is a large B-cell neoplasm that develops in the pleural, pericardial, or peritoneal cavity usually without a detectable tumor mass.[9,17] It is associated with immunodeficiency (HIV) and EBV.[9] Human herpesvirus 8 is present in all cases.[17] Morphologically, the cells have a wide range of appearances, from immunoblastic to anaplastic with large nucleoli.[17] Plasmacytoid differentiation may be seen. Some cells may resemble Reed-Sternberg cells.[9] CD45 is usually expressed, but pan–B-cell markers are lost. The prognosis is extremely poor.

Diffuse large B-cell lymphoma associated with chronic inflammation
DLBCL associated with chronic inflammation is a distinct entity in the 2008 WHO classification. Initially discovered in Japanese patients with artificial pneumothorax for treatment of pulmonary tuberculosis, the term, *pyothorax-associated lymphoma*, was previously used to describe this condition.[18] DLBCL associated with chronic inflammation encompasses a variety of conditions involving chronic inflammation in an enclosed environment, such as metallic implants in bones and joints, chronic osteomyelitis, and surgical mesh implants.[18] This lymphoma often has the morphologic appearance of DLBCL and is associated with EBV.

Lymphomas Involving the Central Nervous System

Primary diffuse large B-cell lymphoma of the central nervous system
DLBCL of the CNS represents all primary intracerebral or intraocular lymphomas.[9] A majority of patients are immunocompetent; incidence is increased with age.[19] The tumors commonly present as solitary, periventricular masses.[20] Histologically, they have an angiocentric pattern of invasion and are positive for B-cell markers by IHC. Lymphoma cells are not seen as a distinct mass; instead, the malignant B cells are seen encircling blood vessels Dissemination to extraneural sites is rare.[9]

Extranodal Plasmacytoma and B-Cell Neoplasms with Plasmacytic Differentiation

Deciding whether a neoplasm is made of pure plasma cells (plasmacytoma) or of B cells with plasmacytic differentiation can be difficult. A plasmacytoma is a neoplasm composed of monoclonal plasma cells that typically involves extranodal tissues. Plasmacytomas do not show evidence of multifocal bone marrow involvement. Also, no clinical or laboratory evidence of myeloma is present. There is a small or absent M-component in urine or serum. There are 2 types of plasmacytomas, including solitary plasmacytoma of bone and extraosseous plasmacytoma. Solitary plasmacytoma of bone consists of a localized single bone tumor composed of plasma cells. Extraosseous plasmacytoma is a neoplasm composed of plasma cells that arises in tissues other than bone. The head and neck area is the most common site in approximately 90% of cases and the GI tract is second most common. By IHC, plasma cells express CD138, CD56, CD38, and MUM1 and is light chain restricted but are CD45 and CD20 negative. Flow cytometry greatly underestimates the number of plasma cells because plasma cells do not flow well. Plasmacytomas show cytogenetic abnormalities similar to plasma cell myeloma. Plasmacytomas may have a hyperploid or nonhyperploid amount of chromosomes. The hyperploid neoplasms have between 48 and 74 chromosomes. Additional translocations include t(11;14), t(4;14), and t(14;16).

Plasmablastic lymphoma
B-cell lymphomas with plasmacytic differentiation are in the pathologic differential diagnosis of

plasmacytoma. Plasmablastic lymphoma is a large B-cell lymphoma with immunoblastic or plasmablastic features and a plasma cell phenotype that has an aggressive clinical course. The oral cavity is the most common site of this lymphoma and approximately 90% of oral cavity plasmablastic lymphomas occur in HIV[+] patients. Nonoral plasmablastic lymphoma is most commonly found in the maxillary sinus and nasopharynx but can be found in any location and commonly in HIV[−] patients. The tumor is composed of large B cells that express morphologic and immunophenotypical features of plasma cells expressing CD138, CD38, and CD79a but usually lacking CD45, CD20, and PAX5.[13] Intermixed with the tumor are varying amounts of benign plasma cells.

Lymphoplasmacytic lymphoma

Lymphoplasmacytic lymphoma (LPL) is within the differential diagnosis of plasmacytoma and plasmablastic lymphoma but only rarely is extranodal. LPL is a neoplasm of small B lymphocytes, with or without plasmacytoid features and plasma cells, that does not meet criteria for any other small B-cell lymphoma showing plasmacytic differentiation. *MYD88* is a gene with a recently discovered mutation that helps differentiate LPL from other lymphomas, including marginal zone lymphoma. The mutation is a result of a single-nucleotide peptide change at position 38182641 on chromosome 3p22.2, causing an amino acid change from leucine to proline (L265P).[21] This mutation can help differentiate LPLs from marginal zone lymphoma because it is mutated in approximately 90% of LPLs and only rarely in marginal zone lymphoma[21] (**Fig. 7**).

Mature T-cell Lymphomas in Extranodal Locations

Enteropathy-associated T-cell lymphoma

EATL is a T-cell lymphoma that is thought to arise from intraepithelial T cells and occurs in the GI tract. There are type 1 and type II EATLs. Type I is usually associated with celiac disease and occurs with higher frequency in northern Europe.[22] Type I EATL is associated with HLA-DQ2/HLA-DQ8 and has a usual immunophenotype of CD3[+], CD4[−], CD8[−], and CD56[−]. Type II EATL is less common than type I and has monomorphic small to medium-sized cells. The immunophenotype is CD3[+], CD4[−], CD8[+], and CD56[+] and has weak to no association with celiac disease. Both types occur in older adults, have frequent presentation of small bowel perforations, spread early to other intra-abdominal sites, lack an association with EBV, and have an aggressive clinical course.[7,22] Type II EATL occurs in all populations with no evidence of racial predilection.[22]

The differential diagnosis of EATL is angioimmunoblastic T-cell lymphoma (AITL). AITL is most commonly nodal based and is thought to derive from follicular helper T cells. These are T cells that are positive for T-cell markers as well as CD10, BCL6, PD1, and CXCL13 (**Fig. 8**).

Hepatosplenic T-cell lymphoma

Hepatosplenic T-cell lymphoma is a sinusoid $\gamma\delta$ T-cell lymphoma found in the splenic red pulp and liver sinusoids and infiltrating the bone marrow. It occurs most commonly in young, immunosuppressed men, most with either a history of organ transplant or Crohn disease and on treatment with tumor necrosis factor α inhibitors. The neoplastic cells are positive for CD56 and cytotoxic markers. CD4 and CD8 are negative. Molecular testing reveals T-cell receptor rearrangement, trisomy 18, and isochromosome 7q. A variant form is from $\alpha\beta$ T cells and has the same morphology, immunophenotype, and genetics but tends to occur in older women.

Extranodal natural killer/T-cell lymphoma, nasal type

Extranodal NK/T-cell lymphoma, nasal type, most commonly occurs in the upper aerodigestive tract, namely the nasal cavity, as the name implies.

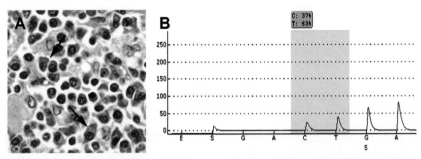

Fig. 7. (*A*) LPL shows plasma cells with eccentrically located nuclei, ample eosinophilic cytoplasm, and peri-nuclear hofs (Hemotoxylin-eosin stain, original magnification, 20×). (*B*) This pyrogram demonstrates the L265 P mutation due to substitution of a T for a C in codon 265 of the *MYD88* gene in a patient with LPL. MYD88 mutations support that a lymphoma is LPL rather than other lymphoma with plasmacytic differentiation, such as marginal zone lymphoma.

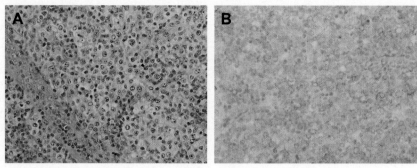

Fig. 8. Morphology and IHC of AITL. (*A*) H&E morphology shows a mass with increased clear lymphocytes. T-cell lymphomas often show increased clear cytoplasm (Hemotoxylin-eosin stain, original magnification, 20×). (*B*) A PD1 IHC stain is positive in the malignant T cells of AITL, which is a marker of follicular helper T-cells (PD1 immunohistochemical stain, original magnification, 20×).

Atypia, necrosis, and angiodestruction are typical features of extranodal NK/T-cell lymphoma, nasal type. Almost all are positive for EBV. The neoplastic cells are positive for CD56 and cytoplasmic CD3. CD4, CD8, and surface CD3 are almost always negative.

SUMMARY

In summary, an overview of the pathology of extranodal lymphoma is presented. The classification system includes B-cell and T-cell lymphomas based on their morphology and phenotype as well as their molecular alterations.

REFERENCES

1. Pileri SA, Agostinelli C, Sabattini E, et al. Lymphoma classification: the quiet after the storm. Semin Diagn Pathol 2011;28(2):113–23.

2. Vasile D, Vladareanu AM, Bumbea H. Peripheral T and NK cell non-hodgkin lymphoma a challenge for diagnosis. J Clin Med 2014;9(1):104–8.

3. Abbas AK, Lichtman AH. Basic immunology: functions and disorders of the immune system. 2nd edition. Saunders; 2004.

4. Restrepo CS, Carrillo J, de Christenson MR, et al. Lymphoproliferative lung disorders: a radiologic-pathologic overview. Part II: neoplastic disorders. Semin Ultrasound CT MR 2013;34(6):535–49.

5. Yu H, Shahsafaei A, Dorfman DM. Germinal-center T-helper-cell markers PD-1 and CXCL13 are both expressed by neoplastic cells in angioimmunoblastic T-cell lymphoma. Am J Clin Pathol 2009;131(1):33–41.

6. Foukas PG, de Leval L. Recent advances in intestinal lymphomas. Histopathology 2015;66:112–36.

7. Peng JC, Zhong L, Ran ZH. Primary lymphomas in the gastrointestinal tract. J Dig Dis 2015;16:169–76.

8. Burke JS. Lymphoproliferative disorders of the gastrointestinal tract. Arch Pathol Lab Med 2011; 135(10):1283–97.

9. Swerdlow SH. WHO classification of tumours of haematopoietic and lymphoid tissues. Lyon (France): International Agency for Research on Cancer; 2008.

10. Meister HP. Malignant lymphomas of soft tissues. Verh Dtsch Ges Pathol 1992;76:140–5.

11. Friedberg JW. Double hit diffuse large B-cell lymphomas: diagnostic and therapeutic challenges. Chin Clin Oncol 2015;4(1):9.

12. Goodlad JR, Fletcher CDM, Chan JKC, et al. Primary soft tissue lymphoma: an analysis of 37 cases. J Pathol 1996;179(Suppl):42A.

13. O'Malley DP, Auerbach A, Weiss LM. Practical applications in immunohistochemistry: evaluation of diffuse large B-cell lymphoma and related large B-cell lymphomas. Arch Pathol Lab Med 2015;139(9):1094–107.

14. Von Beisen K, Kelta M, Bahaguna P. Primary mediastinal B-cell lymphoma: a review of pathology and management. J Clin Oncol 2001;19:1855–64.

15. Parissis H. Forty years literature review of primary lung lymphoma. J Cardiothorac Surg 2011;6:23.

16. Colby TV. Current histological diagnosis of lymphomatoid granulomatosis. Mod Pathol 2012;25:39–42.

17. Kim Y, Park CJ, Roh J, et al. Current concepts in primary effusion lymphoma and other effusion-based lymphomas. Korean J Pathol 2014;48:81–90.

18. Loong F, Chan AC, Ho BC, et al. Diffuse large B-cell lymphoma associated with chronic inflammation as incidental finding and new clinical scenarios. Mod Pathol 2010;23(4):493–501.

19. Phillips EH, Fox CP, Cwynarski K. Primary CNS lymphoma. Curr Hematol Malig Rep 2014;9:243–53.

20. Bhagavathi S, Wilson JD. Primary central nervous system lymphoma. Arch Pathol Lab Med 2008; 132(11):1830–4.

21. Martinez-Lopez A, Curiel-Olmo S, Mollejo M, et al. MYD88 (L265P) somatic mutation in marginal zone B-cell lymphoma. Am J Surg Pathol 2015;39(5):644–51.

22. Chan JKC, Chan ACL, Cheuk W, et al. Type II enteropathy-associated T-cell lymphoma: a distinct aggressive lymphoma with frequent gamma-delta T-cell receptor expression. Am J Surg Pathol 2011; 35:1557–69.

Extranodal Lymphoma of the Central Nervous System and Spine

Kelly K. Koeller, MD[a,b],*, Robert Y. Shih, LTC, MC, USA[b,c,d]

KEYWORDS

- Primary central nervous system lymphoma • Intravascular lymphoma • Lymphomatosis cerebri
- Lymphomatoid granulomatosis • Posttransplantation lymphoproliferative disorder
- Immunosuppression

KEY POINTS

- Central nervous system lymphoma is rare, comprising approximately 6% of all brain tumors.
- Strong affiliation with immunocompromised status is common but it may arise in those with normal immune systems as well.
- Hyperattenuation on computed tomography, mild hypointensity on T2-weighted magnetic resonance imaging, enhancement on postcontrast studies, and periventricular location are characteristic imaging manifestations.
- Less common variant forms include intravascular lymphoma, lymphomatosis cerebri, lymphomatoid granulomatosis, and posttransplantation lymphoproliferative disorder.
- Extranodal lymphoma of the spine is more often caused by secondary dissemination from systemic disease and less often the primary site of origin.

EXTRANODAL LYMPHOMA OF THE CENTRAL NERVOUS SYSTEM

Once an extremely rare brain neoplasm, primary central nervous system lymphoma (PCNSL) and its less common variants now comprise 6% of all primary brain tumors, primarily driven by its firm affiliation with immunocompromised population groups. This single factor and the advent of acquired immunodeficiency syndrome (AIDS) in the late 1970s and early 1980s led to a remarkable surge in prevalence that continued into the early 1990s. For reasons that defy explanation, the prevalence of the disease in the immunocompetent populations groups also increased (albeit to a lesser extent) during this same period.

Because the tumor is known for its dense cellularity and periventricular location, it is often initially characterized on computed tomography (CT) and magnetic resonance (MR) imaging, placing the radiologist on the front line in suggesting the diagnosis and helping guide a multidisciplinary team in management strategies. This article reviews a broad spectrum of clinical, etiologic, and pathologic features that frequently intersect with common radiologic findings of this disease.

PRIMARY CENTRAL NERVOUS SYSTEM LYMPHOMA

PCNSL is a form of extranodal non-Hodgkin lymphoma involving the brain, leptomeninges, spinal

Disclaimer: The opinions and assertions contained herein are the private views of the authors and are not to be construed as official or representing the views of the Departments of the Army or Defense.
[a] Mayo Clinic, Department of Radiology, 200 First Street Southwest, Rochester, MN 55905, USA; [b] American Institute for Radiologic Pathology, Neuroradiology Section, 1010 Wayne Avenue, Suite 320, Silver Spring, MD 20910, USA; [c] Walter Reed National Military Medical Center, Department of Radiology, 8901 Rockville Pike, Bethesda, MD, 20889, USA; [d] Uniformed Services University of the Health Sciences, Department of Radiology, 4301 Jones Bridge Road, Bethesda, MD 20814, USA
* Corresponding author.
E-mail address: koeller.kelly@mayo.edu

Radiol Clin N Am 54 (2016) 649–671
http://dx.doi.org/10.1016/j.rcl.2016.03.003
0033-8389/16/$ – see front matter

cord, or ocular globes.[1] Although still rare, the prevalence of the disease increased substantially during the past 4 decades, with a striking threefold increase between 1973 and 1984, primarily related to the advent of AIDS and the increasing utility of immunosuppression in the setting of solid organ and autologous stem-cell transplantation. This underscores its strong connection for those who are immunocompromised from congenital or acquired immunodeficiency, including those with autoimmune disorders.[1,2] However, its prevalence has also increased among those who are immunocompetent for reasons that are poorly explained. Since a peak in 1993 and in conjunction with the introduction of highly active antiretroviral therapy, the annual incidence of PCNSL has declined in those with AIDS, although its incidence is not significantly changed for those 60 years or older, another higher risk group.[2,3] PCNSL now accounts for approximately 6% of all brain tumors, placing it as the fourth most common primary brain tumor overall.[1,2]

Clinical

Patients with PCNSL present with nonspecific clinical signs and symptoms with a paucity of "B" symptoms (fever, weight loss, and night sweats) so commonly seen in systemic lymphoma. In a multicenter review of 248 patients with primary cerebral lymphoma (96% as PCNSL), most (70%) presented with focal neurologic deficits, whereas neuropsychiatric symptoms (43%), symptoms related to increased intracranial pressure (33%), seizures (14%), and ocular symptoms (4%) were less common.[4] Other studies have shown ocular involvement (commonly with floaters, blurred vision, and painful red eyes) in up to 20% of patients with PCNSL.[1] Accordingly, slit-lamp examination should be included as part of the diagnostic evaluation.[1]

Besides standard neuroimaging (described later in this article), contrast-enhanced CT of the chest, abdomen, and pelvis is recommended in all patients and clinical and ultrasonographic evaluation of the testicles should be considered in older men.[1] As up to 13% of patients with PCNSL have occult extraneural disease, bone marrow biopsy is also recommended.[1]

Cerebrospinal fluid (CSF) analysis plays an important role in the initial and continuing assessment of patients with PCNSL. Increased white blood cell count and protein concentration with lowered CSF glucose levels compared with serum glucose levels are common.[1] Although initial CSF evaluation is often normal, positive cytology is frequently seen on follow-up lumbar punctures.[5]

Prognosis is especially poor for patients with PCNSL who are older than 60 years, have a performance status greater than 1 (Eastern Cooperative Oncology Group performance status scale), elevated serum lactate dehydrogenase (LDH), high CSF protein concentration, and location of the tumor within the deep regions of the brain (periventricular, basal ganglia, brainstem, and/or cerebellum). Those who have 1 to 3 of these features had a 2-year survival rate of 48%, whereas those with 4 to 5 showed only 15% survival rate. In contrast, those patients with none of these parameters had an 80% 2-year survival rate.[6]

Etiology and Pathology

The etiology of PCNSL remains unknown. Several associations beyond immunosuppression have been identified. Epstein-Barr virus (EBV) genome is present in 95% of tumor cells in immunocompromised patients but in fewer than 20% of those with normal immune systems.[2] Some evidence suggests a possible role of the JC virus as a cofactor.[2] Genetic evidence supports the hypothesis that PCNSL is derived from germinal center B cells.[2] Overexpression of numerous genes, most prominently B-cell lymphoma 6 (BCL-6) protein, is linked with PCNSL.[2] This marker is also associated with nearly 7 times longer median survival than those with tumors that did not show expression of this protein.[1]

Whether PCSNL arises in the brain or outside the brain is unresolved. Current hypotheses include development of adhesion molecules on transformed B cells outside the brain, preservation of lymphoma cells in the brain as a "safe haven," and expansion of a polyclonal inflammatory lesion in the brain into a monoclonal state.[2] Historically, the brain has been recognized for its lack of a classic lymphatic drainage system and fueled controversy regarding the histogenesis of PCNSL in such a structure. Recently, Louveau and colleagues[7] reported the discovery of functional lymphatic vessels lining the dural sinuses that has altered this perspective and other assumptions about neuroimmunology.

On gross pathology, the tumor shows frequent but not invariable demarcation from normal brain with most lesions occupying a periventricular location (**Fig. 1**E). More diffuse involvement of the brain, as is typical in glial neoplasms, also may be seen but is less conspicuous.[2] Single lesions are reported in 66% of cases overall but multiple lesions share nearly equal prevalence in the immunocompromised and tend to show more necrosis than in the immunocompetent population.[2,8]

Nearly all (95%) of PCNSLs are classified as diffuse large B-cell lymphoma (DLBCL) and express characteristic immunohistochemical markers for that cell lineage, such as CD19 and

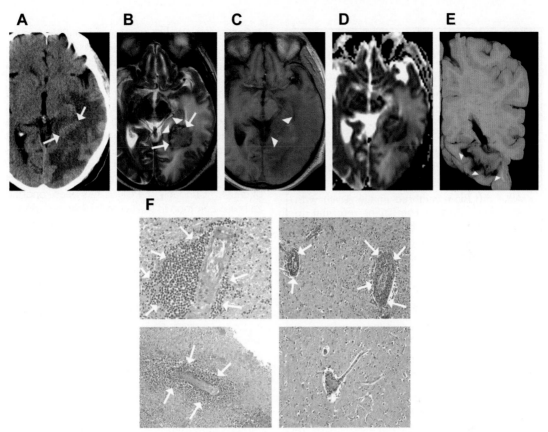

Fig. 1. CNS lymphoma in an immunocompromised adult with prior liver transplantation and recent onset of headaches and disorientation. (*A*) Axial noncontrast CT image shows ill-defined hyperattenuation (*arrows*) of the left periatrial region. (*B*) Axial T2W MR image reveals hypointensity and better definition of the mass (*arrows*) compared with surrounding vasogenic edema. Peripheral more prominent hypointensity (*arrowheads*) likely reflects hemorrhage. (*C*) Axial T1W MR image reveals hypointensity with subtle peripheral hyperintensity (*arrowheads*) that again likely reflects hemorrhage. (*D*) Axial apparent diffusion coefficient MR image reveals corresponding hypointensity of the mass, representing restricted diffusion. (*E*) Coronal photograph of gross postmortem specimen shows correlative mass (*arrows*) along inferior margin of left atrium. Hemorrhagic rim (*arrowheads*) corresponds to T2W and T1W imaging findings. (*F*) Histopathology showed DLBCL in context of posttransplantation lymphoproliferative disorder. Montage of 4 photomicrographs (hematoxylin and eosin stain, low magnification) demonstrates extensive perivascular lymphocytes (*arrows*).

CD20.[2] The remaining 5% are composed of low-grade lymphomas corresponding to their systemic counterparts, including lymphoplasmocytic lymphoma, mucosa-associated lymphoid tissue (MALT) lymphoma, and marginal zone B-cell lymphoma (MZBCL). The MALT lymphoma and MZBCL usually manifest as a dural-based mass that often mimics a meningioma on gross pathologic and neuroradiologic examination.[2] T-cell PCNSL (T-PCNSL) is more common in Asian countries, comprising 8% to 14% of PCNSL in Japan and 17% in Korea compared with 2% to 5% in Western countries.[9] These findings also match the generally increased incidence of other T-cell lymphomas in Asian population groups.[9,10] Hodgkin lymphoma is rare (0.2%–0.5%) in the central nervous system (CNS) and nearly always occurs in the presence of grade III or IV systemic disease

(regarded as secondary CNS lymphoma).[2] This lymphoma has a predilection for a dural location but may also arise within the brain parenchyma.[2,11]

The lymphocytes of PCNSL have a distinct predilection for the perivascular spaces, creating clusters of lymphoid material with densely packed cells that are noteworthy for a high nucleus-to-cytoplasm ratio (**Fig. 1**F). Although predominantly composed of B-cell lymphocytes, occasional T-cell lymphocytes are also present but are believed to simply represent a reactive process.[2]

Neuroimaging

The combination of a periventricular location and dense cellularity of the tumor represents a characteristic imaging appearance for PCNSL (**Boxes 1 and 2**). On CT, a mildly hyperattenuated mass in

Solitary lesions are more common (65% in a review of 100 immunocompetent patients with PCNSL) than those that are multifocal.[5] However, multifocal disease is more commonly seen in the immunocompromised setting, as is necrosis.[5,8] The cerebral hemisphere is the most common site whereas approximately a third of lesions arise in the deep gray matter.[8] Bulky infiltration of the corpus callosum is considered a highly characteristic imaging manifestation of the disease (**Fig. 3**).[5] Cerebellar lesions are noted in approximately 10% of cases.[8] Curiously, T-PCNSL has been reported as more common in the posterior fossa in reports from Western countries, but this finding has not been corroborated in reports from Asian countries.[9,10,12,13]

"Sentinel lesions" have been reported in small groups of patients with nonspecific clinical presentations and initial identification of small focal enhancing lesions in the brain that either spontaneously regress or, more commonly, resolve following the administration of corticosteroid therapy.[14,15] This may support the polyclonal-monoclonal hypothesis described earlier as an explanation for histogenesis.[2]

Intraventricular involvement is uncommon (11.8% in the series of 100 immunocompetent patients).[5] Leptomeningeal disease is estimated at 20% but may be underestimated, as this may be difficult to confidently identify on MR imaging.[5] In distinction to PCNSL, the much less common T-PCNSLs usually occur in superficial or subcortical regions of the cerebral hemispheres and usually with rim enhancement on postcontrast imaging.[9]

Magnetic resonance spectroscopy has been reported to show changes in major metabolic peaks typical for a brain tumor but are not specific for

---

Box 1
Simplified imaging protocols

Computed tomography (CT) imaging protocol

- Unenhanced CT to identify hyperattenuated parenchymal masses

Magnetic resonance (MR) imaging protocol

- Sagittal T1-weighted (T1W)
- Axial T2 fluid-attenuated inversion recovery to assess for vasogenic edema
- Axial diffusion-weighted image (DWI) with apparent diffusion coefficient reformat to assess for restricted diffusion
- Axial T2-weighted (T2W) to assess for mild hypointensity compared with surrounding edema
- Precontrast axial T1W
- Postcontrast axial and coronal T1W
- (Optional) Gradient-recalled echo or susceptibility-weighted imaging
- (Optional) Perfusion imaging

---

the periventricular region is common, whereas it is mildly hypointense on T2-weighted (T2W) MR imaging compared with more prominent and hyperintense vasogenic edema. MR T1-weighted (T1W) images show hypointensity compared with more conspicuous surrounding hypointensity that correlates with vasogenic edema. The overwhelming majority of PCNSL lesions showing intense enhancement on postcontrast techniques with both CT and MR imaging (**Figs. 1** and **2**).[8] Enhancement is more commonly ringlike in those arising in immunocompromised patients.[8]

Box 2
Characteristic imaging findings of primary central nervous system lymphoma (PCNSL)

Modality	Features
CT	
Unenhanced	Hyperattenuated
Contrast-enhanced	Enhanced
MR imaging	
T1W	Isointense-to-hypointense
T2W	Mildly hypointense compared to surrounding edema
DWI	Hyperintense (restricted diffusion)
Contrast-enhanced T1W	Often intense enhancement, ring-like in immunocompromised
Metabolic	
PET (fluorodeoxyglucose, methionine) and	Hypermetabolic
Single-photon emission computed tomography (SPECT) (thallium)	

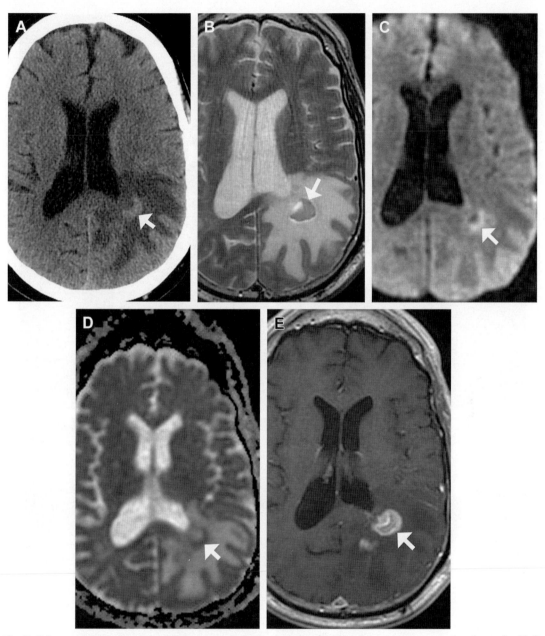

Fig. 2. Primary CNS lymphoma. (*A*) Noncontrast CT image shows focal nodular hyperattenuation (*arrow*) of left periatrial white matter. (*B*) Axial T2W MR image demonstrates mild hypointensity of the mass (*arrow*) compared with more prominent hyperintensity of presumed surrounding vasogenic edema. (*C*) Axial DWI shows curvilinear hyperintensity (*arrow*). (*D*) Corresponding axial apparent diffusion coefficient MR image reveals hypointensity (*arrow*), consistent with restricted diffusion. (*E*) Contrast-enhanced axial T1W MR image demonstrates associated intense enhancement (*arrow*). Histopathology showed diffuse large B-cell lymphoma.

PCNSL. Decreased n-acetyl aspartate and creatine with markedly elevated choline, lactic acid, and lipids/macromolecules is common. Myo-inositol is usually normal or mildly decreased.[5]

Metabolic imaging is valuable for distinguishing PCNSL from other neoplasms and from toxoplasmosis. Fluorodeoxyglucose PET (FDG-PET) and 11C-methionine PET both typically depict increased metabolic activity of PCNSL compared with

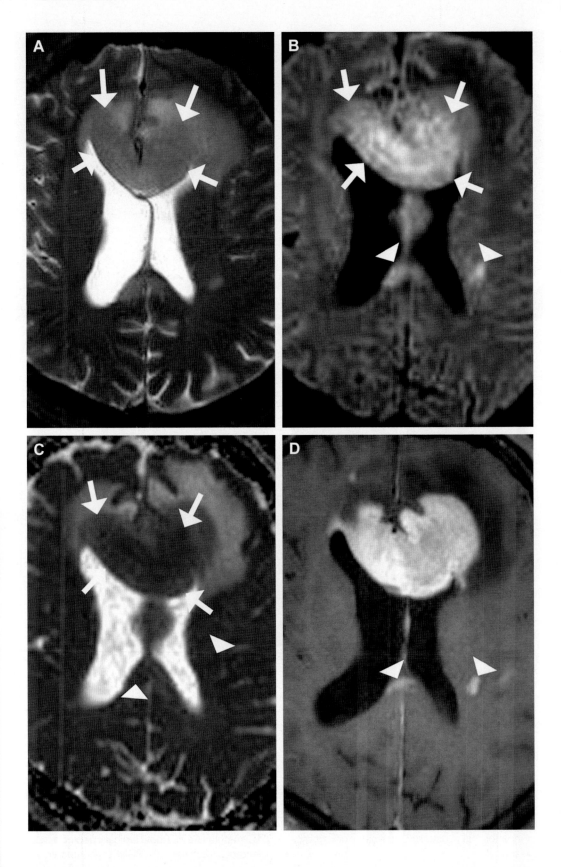

infectious etiologies such as toxoplasmosis (**Fig. 4**). 11C-methionine PET often shows very high uptake in PCNSL beyond the enhancing margin seen on MR imaging, presumably reflecting infiltration, and may increase accuracy in establishing the true size of the tumor. In immunocompromised patients, thallium-201 single-photon emission computed tomography (SPECT) is effective for differentiating PCNSL from toxoplasmosis.[16]

Making a distinction of toxoplasmosis, the most common cause of an intracranial mass in the immunocompromised adult, from PCNSL, the next most common cause, is of prime importance because of marked differences in therapy and prognosis for the 2 diseases. Although this has traditionally been established through an empiric 2-week trial of antitoxoplasmosis therapy (with decreasing size of the toxoplasmosis lesions), the impact of such a delay in a patient with PCNSL, with such a guarded prognosis, cannot be understated. The potential identification of PCNSL through PET or SPECT can markedly accelerate the diagnostic evaluation and initiation of appropriate therapy without a delay of 2 or more weeks using an empiric trial. Glioma, demyelinating disease, other infections, and vascular diseases may share some similar imaging features with PCNSL (**Boxes 3 and 4**).[8]

Treatment

A stereotactic biopsy is indicated for all patients with clinical, laboratory, and neuroimaging findings suggesting the diagnosis of PCNSL.[1] Surgical resection alone is inadequate for treatment and survival (median of only 1–4 months in that setting).[1,17]

Although an initial positive response to corticosteroid therapy is often seen in PCNSL, enlargement of the tumor and increased associated edema invariably returns a short while later. Even more significant is the well-documented interference with establishing the histopathologic diagnosis of the tumor after corticosteroid therapy

has been administered. Therefore, this therapy should be withheld until the biopsy has been completed if at all possible.[1,18]

Radiation therapy, once used as a frontline therapy, suffers from limited efficacy (median survival of only 12–18 months) and significant risk of delayed neurotoxicity, especially in patients older than 60 years. It is now primarily reserved as an adjunct to multiagent chemotherapy or for the setting of chemotherapeutic failure.[1]

Methotrexate-based multiagent chemotherapy is regarded as the initial therapy of choice in the management of patients with PCNSL, particularly for patients older than 60 years.[1] In one study, combination methotrexate and cytarabine therapy effected a 5-year survival rate of 75% for those younger than 60 years and an overall survival of 34% in those older than 60 years.[19] Even better outcomes, particularly in patients younger than 65 years, have been achieved with combination high-dose chemotherapy and autologous stem-cell transplantation, up to 87% 5-year survival with adjunct whole brain radiation therapy.[20,21] More recently, the addition of rituximab to standard chemotherapy led to 78% 3-year survival compared with only 40% for those who did receive this monoclonal antibody agent.[22] The development of more effective chemotherapeutic protocols remains an area of intense investigation.[1]

INTRAVASCULAR LYMPHOMA

In 1959, 2 Austrian dermatologists, Josef Tappeiner and Lilly Pfleger, were the first to publish a case report of an unusual proliferative multilocular disease within the vascular endothelium causing thrombosis and occlusion.[23,24] In subsequent reports, it became clear there were 2 distinct and diametrically opposed subgroups: one as a benign self-limited reactive inflammatory process and the other as an extremely aggressive malignant neoplasm spreading beyond the vessels and that was fatal within 2 years of onset.[23,25,26]

Fig. 3. Primary CNS lymphoma. (*A*) Axial T2W MR image reveals mildly hyperintense corpus callosal mass centered in the genu of the corpus callosum with prominent surrounding hyperintensity, most consistent with vasogenic edema. The mass is slightly hypointense compared with surrounding vasogenic edema, a characteristic imaging manifestation of this tumor. Smaller areas (*arrowheads*) of hyperintensity are seen in the left centrum semiovale and splenium of the corpus callosum. (*B*) Axial diffusion-weighted MR image shows corresponding hyperintensity of the mass (*arrows*) and smaller lesions (*arrowheads*). (*C*) Axial apparent diffusion coefficient MR image reveals corresponding hypointensity (*arrows and arrowheads*), confirming restricted diffusion. (*D*) Contrast-enhanced axial T1W MR image demonstrates intense enhancement of the mass. Focal enhancement (*arrowheads*) corresponds to smaller regions of FLAIR/T2 hyperintensity of the left centrum semiovale and splenium of the corpus callosum, representing additional involvement. Excisional biopsy was performed and showed diffuse large B-cell lymphoma on histopathology. (*Courtesy of* David Black, MD, Mayo Clinic, Rochester, MN.)

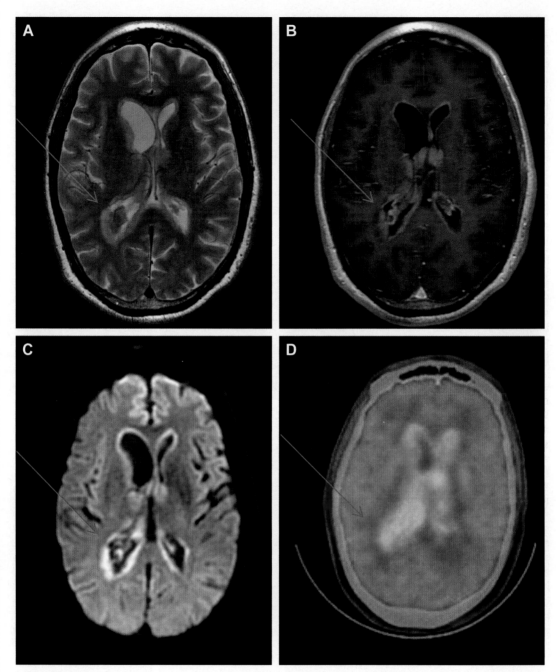

Fig. 4. A 58-year-old man with progressive cognitive and gait dysfunction from primary CNS lymphoma. (*A*) Axial T2W and (*B*) postgadolinium images reveal abnormal nodular enhancement along the ventricular margin, most advanced at the right atrium (*red arrows*). (*C*) Diffusion-weighted and (*D*) fused FDG-PET/CT images confirm hypercellularity and hypermetabolism, respectively. Surgical biopsy was consistent with DLBCL.

Decades later, subsequent immunohistochemical investigations revealed this neoplasm as a lymphoma and, in 2008, the World Health Organization (WHO) classified it as intravascular large B-cell lymphoma (IVL), also known as angiotropic lymphoma.[2]

Most cases of IVL arise in patients of older age (median age of 70 years). A previous or concomitant malignancy is noted in 16%.[27] Similar to cases of PCNSL, the clinical presentation is nonspecific with fever without or with B symptoms (45%). A spectrum of skin lesions has been

Box 3
Simplified differential diagnosis

Neoplastic Disease

- Glioma (more commonly higher grade, such as glioblastoma multiforme)
- Metastasis
- Primitive neuroectodermal tumor (primarily in children)

Infectious Disease

- Abscess (especially toxoplasmosis in immuno-compromised patients)
- Sarcoidosis
- Tuberculosis
- Other granulomatous diseases

Demyelinating Disease

- Multiple sclerosis (enhancing active plaques; periventricular location)

Vascular Disease

- Vasculitis

sized vessels, causing thrombosis and occlusion and leading to infarction.[2]

Neuroimaging, particularly MR imaging, reveals correlative evidence of these ischemic changes on occasion, although it may be falsely negative in some cases.[27] Multifocal lesions are far more common than a single lesion.[28] Restricted diffusion on diffusion-weighted imaging (DWI) and associated fluid-attenuated inversion recovery (FLAIR)/T2 hyperintensity and T1 hypointensity is frequently noted.[28,29] In addition, cerebral masses may also be noted and conform to the pattern for PCNSL described previously.[28–30] Enhancement is commonly seen, although not universal, and may involve the meninges as well as the parenchyma (**Figs. 5** and **6**).[28] Dural sinus thrombosis related to lymphomatous invasion has also been reported.[31]

Although not as bleak as reported in Tappeiner and Pfleger's original article,[27] the prognosis for IVL remains poor with a 22% 3-year survival rate reported in 2004. Anthracycline-based chemotherapy, supplemented by autologous stem-cell transplantation, is commonly used but progression and recurrences are common.[27] The one exception is in the setting of the "cutaneous variant," in which the skin is the only site of involvement and which has occurred nearly exclusively in women of a slightly younger age and with a much better outlook. For those with a single skin lesion, limited radiotherapy to the site may suffice with long-term survival.[27] Conversely, the "Asian variant," known for a prominent hemophagocytic syndrome, bone marrow involvement,

reported, including painful erythematous eruption, violaceous plaques, "peau d'orange" appearance, and other manifestations.[27] Although virtually any solid organ may be involved, the CNS (39%) and skin (40%) are the most common sites.[2,27] Serum LDH levels are typically elevated.[27] Histopathological review demonstrates predominantly B-cell lymphocytes accumulating in small and medium-

Box 4
Pearls and pitfalls

Pearls

- Single lesion more common (66%) overall, whereas multiple lesions and necrotic lesions are more common in the immunocompromised.
- Hyperattenuated (CT) and hypointense (T2W MR) periventricular mass is typical.
- Basal ganglia and corpus callosum involvement characteristic.
- Curvilinear enhancement characteristic for intravascular involvement (intravascular lymphoma; frequently with dementia).

Pitfalls

- Toxoplasmosis may mimic appearance in immunocompromised. Antitoxoplasmosis therapy trial or metabolic imaging (PET, SPECT) may clarify.
- Glioblastoma multiforme is other common neoplasm to cross corpus callosum ("butterfly glioma").
- "Ghost tumor" with steroid therapy: lesion may resolve quickly and interfere with histopathologic diagnosis on stereotactic biopsy.
- Secondary central nervous system lymphoma more commonly involves dura rather than brain parenchyma and may mimic meningioma.

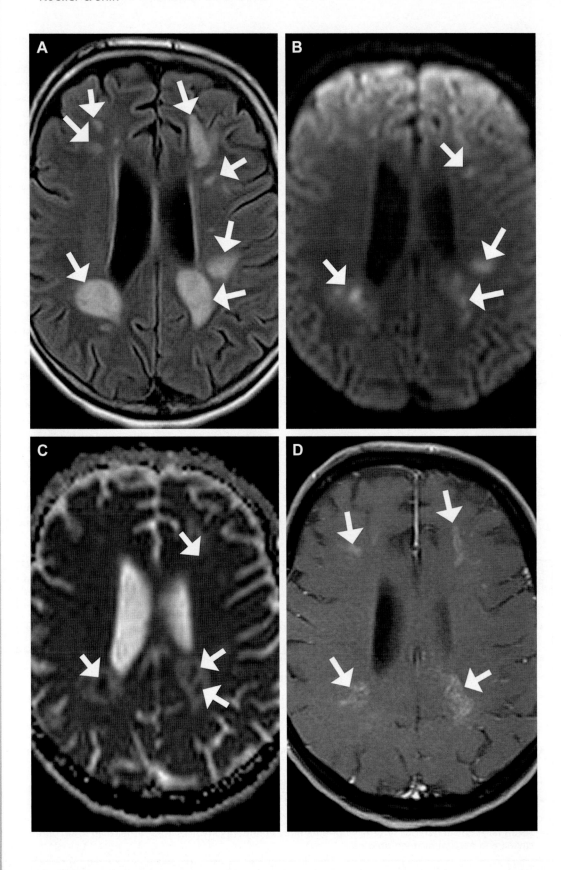

hepatosplenomegaly, and thrombocytopenia but less common involvement of the CNS, is even more biologically aggressive than IVL with a median survival of only 2 to 8 months.[32]

LYMPHOMATOSIS CEREBRI

Lymphomatosis cerebri is a rare variant of PCNSL with diffuse infiltration of the cerebral white matter by lymphoma cells without a well-defined mass. From a few case reports in the literature, the disease presents in patients with a mean age of 64 years (range 41–76 years).[33,34] Rapidly progressive dementia, abnormal gait, focal weakness, and severe weight loss are common clinical features. Orthostatic hypotension has been noted in one case.[33] The prognosis is dismal, with most cases fatal within 6 months of presentation.[34] Early tissue diagnosis and treatment with corticosteroids and radiation therapy have been anecdotally linked with longer survival but optimal treatment remains unknown.[33,34]

Neuroimaging studies reveal absence of a discrete intracranial mass. CT findings are usually minimal without altered attenuation. MR imaging typically shows a highly nonspecific pattern with ill-defined FLAIR/T2 hyperintensity within the cerebral white matter with minimal associated mass effect. Involvement of the cerebral subcortical white matter extending to the deep gray matter structures and brainstem is common. DWI commonly shows no altered signal intensity to suggest restricted diffusion. Postcontrast MR imaging may reveal subtle enhancement, but most lesions do not enhance.[34] FDG-PET scans may show some regional hypermetabolism, although, as with gliomatosis cerebri, normal metabolic activity is common.[34] Histopathologic findings may be clarified with immunohistochemical stains revealing the true nature of the lymphoma cell infiltration.[34] The combination of nonspecific clinical and imaging findings may lead to confusion for Binswanger dementia and a wide range of infectious, inflammatory, vascular, toxic, and neurodegenerative diseases and often leads to a delay in establishing the correct diagnosis.[35,36]

LYMPHOMATOID GRANULOMATOSIS

Lymphomatoid granulomatosis (LG) is a very rare EBV-driven angiocentric and angiodestructive lymphoproliferative process that occurs most prominently in the lung. Involvement of the CNS is reported to occur in up to 20% of cases and is nearly always in association with pulmonary disease. Men are involved more commonly by a 2:1 ratio. The disease presents most commonly in the fourth to sixth decades.[37] Common clinical presentations include confusion, ataxia, hemiparesis, seizures, and cranial neuropathies.[38]

Neuroimaging studies have revealed a wide spectrum of imaging manifestations. In a review of 25 patients with MR imaging from the National Institutes of Health, Patsalides and colleagues[39] reported that nearly half had normal studies. Multifocal parenchymal lesions with FLAIR/T2 hyperintensity of the hemispheric white matter, deep gray matter, or the brainstem were the most common abnormal imaging manifestations and often accompanied with punctate or linear enhancement that was believed to characteristically correlate with perivascular and vascular wall infiltration related to the disease process. Leptomeningeal and cranial nerve enhancement was the next most common. Less commonly, focal masses, dural enhancement, and choroid plexus engorgement were also documented.[39] Contrary to an earlier primarily CT-based study, no frank hemorrhages or predilection for the posterior fossa were identified.[39,40]

Definitive therapeutic protocols in the management of LG remain elusive. Some investigators use the disease grade, determined by the proportion of large atypical EBV-positive B-cells and necrosis compared with the reactive background of T lymphocytes, to guide therapy with interferon-alpha used for immune-dependent grade I and II disease and immunochemotherapy (including rituximab) for immune-independent grade III disease.[37] A positive response of CNS disease to interferon therapy is common for grade I and II disease, although relapse with high-grade disease is possible. The outlook is more guarded for grade III disease.[37]

Fig. 5. Intravascular lymphoma. (*A*) Axial FLAIR MR image shows multiple hyperintense nodular areas (*arrows*) of bilateral hemispheric white matter. (*B*) Axial diffusion-weighted MR image reveals hyperintensity (*arrows*) of these lesions. (*C*) Axial apparent diffusion coefficient MR image demonstrates corresponding hypointensity (*arrows*), indicative of restricted diffusion. (*D*) Contrast-enhanced axial T1W MR image reveals corresponding enhancement (*arrows*) of these lesions. Curvilinear enhancement pattern of left frontal lesion suggests vascular involvement. Histopathology following stereotactic biopsy of right parietal lesion revealed intravascular large B-cell lymphoma associated with subacute infarct on histopathology.

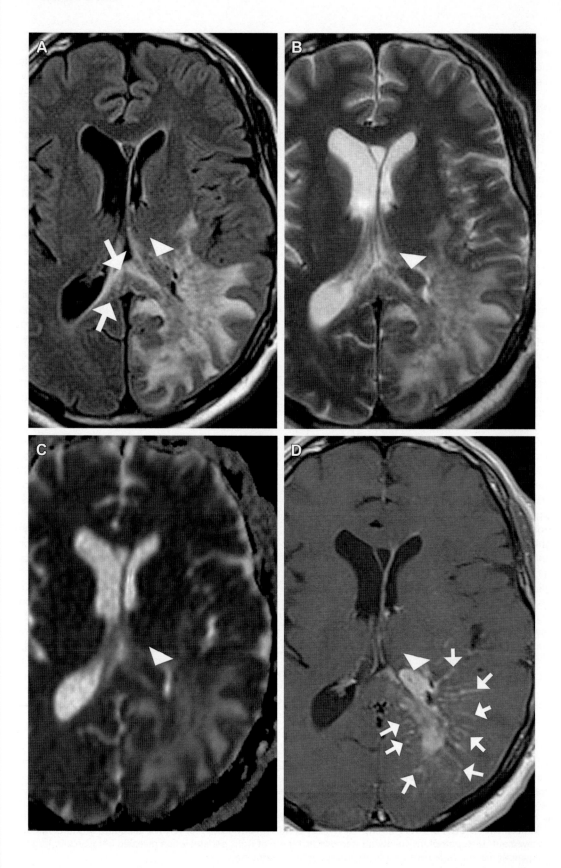

POSTTRANSPLANT LYMPHOPROLIFERATIVE DISORDER

Posttransplant lymphoproliferative disorder (PTLD) is a rare serious complication following solid organ transplantation or bone marrow allografts in immunosuppressed recipients.[41,42] The disorder is caused by a rapid proliferation of lymphocytes, with most cases related to B-cell lymphocytes. EBV has been identified as a causative factor in 90% of cases.[41] The overall incidence of PTLD is estimated at less than 2% of all transplantation cases.[42] Among immunosuppressive agents affiliated with PTLD, cyclosporine and tacrolimus are reported most frequently, although this association may simply reflect their common usage rather than a statistically significant factor.[41]

PTLD is classified by the WHO into 3 categories: early lesions, polymorphic PTLD, and monomorphic PTLD.[43] Reactive plasmacytic hyperplasia characterizes the early lesions and is associated with a mononucleosislike illness. Polymorphic PTLD comprises atypical lymphoid infiltrates consisting of both polyclonal and monoclonal cells. Monomorphic PTLD represents lymphomas (B-cell, T-cell, Burkitt, Hodgkin) and myeloma.[43]

Involvement of the CNS in PTLD is uncommon, with a reported incidence of 15% but varies with the type of solid organ being transplanted, as high as 27% following pancreas transplantation to 13% in lung recipients.[44] Of those patients with CNS PTLD, nearly half have isolated CNS involvement.[44] Nearly all reported CNS PTLD cases are of the monomorphic type and most of this type would be classified as large B-cell lymphomas under the revised European-American lymphoma classification.[42]

On neuroimaging studies, multiple lesions are more common (61%–83%) and with a predilection for the periventricular/basal ganglia region.[41] A posterior fossa location is noted in 4% to 33% of cases.[41,42] On CT, lesions are usually isoattenuated to hyperattenuated compared with the surrounding brain, presumably reflecting hypercellularity.[45] On MR imaging, lesions are usually isointense to hypointense on T1W images with occasional hyperintensity believed to represent areas of hemorrhage.[45] Hypointensity on T2W images is typical and likely related to hypercellularity.[45] Postcontrast MR imaging shows frequent associated enhancement, either homogeneous (41%) or ringlike (29%) (**Fig. 7**).[41,45] Rare spontaneous regression of histologically proven PTLD has been reported.[46]

Initial therapy is directed at reduction of immunosuppression, although the response is variable. Polymorphic PTLD often responds well, whereas monomorphic PTLD may respond more modestly.[41,47] Subsequent therapy focuses on chemotherapy (especially methotrexate) and radiation therapy with some consideration of antiviral medications.[41] More recently, monoclonal antibody therapy with rituximab has also shown promise in patients who do not respond adequately to more conventional interventions.[41]

The prognosis for patients with PTLD with CNS involvement remains poor. In one study, only 9% of adults and 13% of children were still living at 3 years.[44] Children with isolated CNS involvement had better survival compared with those with multisite disease.[44] Originally reported survival rates were lower than that seen in PCNSL. However, a median survival of 47 months has been documented more recently and more closely approximates that of PCNSL in immunocompetent patients.[41] Longer survival periods in those with CNS PTLD compared with other forms of PCNSL have been noted in some cases.[42]

EXTRANODAL LYMPHOMA OF THE SPINE

Like other neoplastic diseases of the spine, extranodal lymphoma of the spine is more often caused by secondary dissemination from extraspinal disease, and less often the primary site of origin. Primary or secondary involvement of the spine is more often associated with non-Hodgkin lymphoma, especially the diffuse large B-cell subtype,

Fig. 6. Primary CNS lymphoma (MALT lymphoma). (*A*) Axial FLAIR MR image shows a nodular mass (*arrowhead*) along the left periatrial margin with prominent heterogeneous hyperintensity of surrounding white matter consistent with vasogenic edema. Abnormal hyperintensity is also seen within the splenium of the corpus callosum (*arrows*). (*B*) Axial T2W MR image reveals better visualization of the nodular mass (*arrowhead*). (*C*) Axial apparent diffusion coefficient MR image demonstrates corresponding hypointensity (*arrowhead*), indicative of restricted diffusion. (*D*) Contrast-enhanced axial T1W MR image shows intense enhancement of the nodular mass (*arrowhead*) and prominent curvilinear enhancement (*small arrows*) within the surrounding white matter, suggesting vascular extension. Although not specific, such a curvilinear appearance is regarded as highly characteristic for CNS lymphoma. Histopathology from stereotactic biopsy revealed low-grade B-cell lymphoma with plasmacytic differentiation consistent with MALT lymphoma.

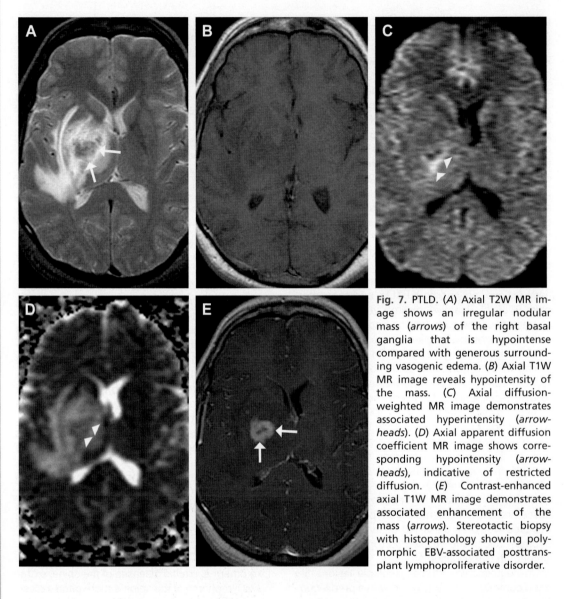

Fig. 7. PTLD. (*A*) Axial T2W MR image shows an irregular nodular mass (*arrows*) of the right basal ganglia that is hypointense compared with generous surrounding vasogenic edema. (*B*) Axial T1W MR image reveals hypointensity of the mass. (*C*) Axial diffusion-weighted MR image demonstrates associated hyperintensity (*arrowheads*). (*D*) Axial apparent diffusion coefficient MR image shows corresponding hypointensity (*arrowheads*), indicative of restricted diffusion. (*E*) Contrast-enhanced axial T1W MR image demonstrates associated enhancement of the mass (*arrows*). Stereotactic biopsy with histopathology showing polymorphic EBV-associated posttransplant lymphoproliferative disorder.

and less often associated with Hodgkin lymphoma, except in the setting of advanced or relapsed disease. Because lymphomas are highly sensitive to radiation and chemotherapy, including corticosteroids, surgical intervention is usually reserved for diagnostic biopsy, fracture stabilization, or cord decompression. Like other spinal neoplasms, spinal lymphomas may be categorized according to their site of origin by anatomic compartment, which are listed in decreasing order of frequency: vertebral, extradural, and intradural lymphomas.[48]

LYMPHOMA OF THE VERTEBRAL COLUMN

Common malignancies of the vertebral column include metastatic disease, multiple myeloma, and disseminated lymphoma. Primary lymphoma of bone, including the vertebral column, is rare and accounts for less than 5% of extranodal lymphomas, and less than 1% of non-Hodgkin lymphomas. The age range is broad, with peak incidence at approximately 60 years, and there is slight male predominance. The most common histologic subtype is diffuse large B-cell lymphoma, which accounts for 70% to 80% of cases.[49] According to most reviews, primary bone lymphoma involves the long bones, particularly the metaphysis or diaphysis of the femur, more frequently than the spinal column. One large series from British Columbia found a higher proportion of primary vertebral lymphoma, with approximately one-third of cases each in the spinal column, in the long bones, and in the flat bones.[50]

Primary or secondary vertebral lymphoma may present with local pain, mass effect, or as an incidental radiologic finding. Mass effect may result from pathologic fracture or epidural spread and may present with myelopathy or radiculopathy. Unlike metastatic carcinoma and solid malignancies, diffuse large B-cell lymphoma usually responds to R-CHOP (rituximab, cyclophosphamide, doxorubicin, vincristine, prednisolone) chemotherapy within days rather than weeks, so retrospective studies have differed on whether surgical intervention is beneficial or needed in patients with cord compression.[51,52] In this setting, another option is combined modality therapy with chemotherapy plus adjuvant radiation. Although studies have shown added benefit from rituximab, a monoclonal antibody against CD20 on B cells, there is no clear consensus on combined modality therapy versus chemotherapy alone.[49]

The radiographic appearance of vertebral lymphoma is variable, but most often osteolytic with either a permeative or moth-eaten pattern of destruction, which may be explained by the presence of osteoclast-stimulating factor.[53] Some other aggressive radiographic features are cortical breakthrough, extraosseous soft tissue mass, and lamellated or interrupted periosteal reaction.[54] Pathologic fracture may cause varying degrees of height loss, ultimately culminating in vertebra plana. These findings are nonspecific and can be seen with other lymphoproliferative disorders, such as leukemia and myeloma, other bone malignancies, such as Ewing sarcoma and osteosarcoma, and inflammatory conditions, such as tuberculous spondylitis and Langerhans cell histiocytosis.[55] Presence of a sequestrum or crossing of discs/joints are more unique findings, which can be seen in lymphoma or infection (Figs. 8 and 9).[56,57]

The presence of systemic or B symptoms may further complicate the differential diagnosis of lymphoma versus infection. There are multiple case reports in the literature of primary vertebral and paravertebral lymphoma being mistaken for an infectious process, especially tuberculous spondylitis, due to the presence of fever, night sweats, and weight loss.[58,59] One case report of primary vertebral lymphoma in the thoracic spine presented with fever, back pain, and elevated inflammatory markers, then underwent open biopsy and decompressive surgery for myelopathy, with histologic diagnosis of chronic inflammatory cell infiltrate, and clinical diagnosis of presumed mycobacterial infection. A CT-guided biopsy of a new anterior mediastinal mass 6 months later revealed Reed-Sternberg cells and a true diagnosis of extranodal Hodgkin lymphoma originating in the thoracic spine.[60]

Hodgkin lymphoma is less likely to arise from an extranodal site than non-Hodgkin lymphoma (approximately 10% vs 40%) and is more likely to elicit reactive osteoblastic or sclerotic changes in the spine, ultimately culminating in the ivory vertebra sign (Fig. 10).[61] On MR imaging, both Hodgkin and non-Hodgkin lymphomas are low signal intensity on T1-weighted images from marrow replacement, variable signal intensity on T2-weighted images depending on the fibrous content, and demonstrate enhancement.[62] Extension from the marrow space into the paraspinal-epidural soft tissues may occur without cortical bone destruction, via small penetrating channels or tumor tunnels.[63] With regard to nuclear imaging, FDG-PET is more sensitive and specific than bone scintigraphy (see Fig. 8) and is recommended for the staging of aggressive and potentially curable lymphomas (eg, diffuse large B-cell and Hodgkin).[64,65]

LYMPHOMA OF THE EXTRADURAL SPACE

Mass lesions of the epidural space usually arise by local extension from the vertebral column, whether degenerative (eg, herniation) or neoplastic (eg, metastasis). Other routes into the epidural space include the neural foramina for paraspinal masses (eg, neurogenic tumor) and hematogenous dissemination. It is uncommon for neoplasms, including lymphoma, to arise within the epidural compartment. A diagnosis of primary spinal epidural lymphoma requires isolated nondisseminated disease and comprises fewer than 1% of extranodal lymphomas.[66] Although some cases may actually reflect local or hematogenous spread from unidentified disease sites, resulting in a false diagnosis of primary rather than secondary epidural lymphoma, other cases have been hypothesized to arise directly from rests of lymphoid tissue that coexist along with venous plexus in the epidural space.[67,68]

Primary spinal epidural lymphoma shares many of the same clinical and histologic features as primary bone lymphoma involving the vertebral column. Peak incidence occurs in middle-aged adults, older than 40 years, although the age range is broad and does include children.[69,70] Male individuals are affected more often than female individuals. Patients can experience localized back pain or radiculopathy, whereas systemic B symptoms or myelopathy is more typical of advanced disease.[71] The thoracic spine is most commonly involved, which may be due to the longer territory, or the more extensive venous

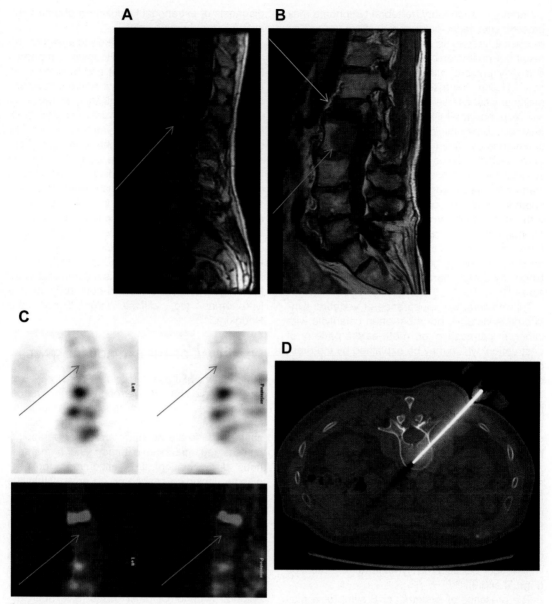

Fig. 8. A 64-year-old asymptomatic man with primary bone lymphoma of the lumbar spine. (*A*) Sagittal T1W images from 2006 and (*B*) from 2013 reveal a slowly enlarging hypointense lesion in the L2 vertebral body (*red arrow*) and interval vertebroplasty at L1 (*green arrow*). The lesion was hyperintense on T2W images with postcontrast enhancement (not shown). (*C*) The lesion was also invisible on bone scan and CT (*blue arrow*), then hypermetabolic on subsequent PET (not shown). (*D*) CT-guided core needle biopsy was diagnostic of a follicular lymphoma, which is the most common low-grade or indolent non-Hodgkin lymphoma.

plexus.[72] Many histologic subtypes of lymphoma have been reported in the epidural space, although overall non-Hodgkin is more common than Hodgkin, and within non-Hodgkin lymphoma, high-grade B-cell tumors are more common than either low-grade B-cell or T-cell lymphomas.[68]

As expected, plain radiography has limited utility for the evaluation of primary spinal epidural lymphoma. MRI with or without gadolinium is the modality of choice for soft tissue evaluation within the spinal canal, including the epidural space. For patients with contraindications to MRI, alternatives include CT or myelography. On MRI, epidural lymphoma is more often dorsal than ventral in location, with low signal intensity on T1-weighted images from fat replacement, variable signal intensity on T2-weighted images, and postcontrast

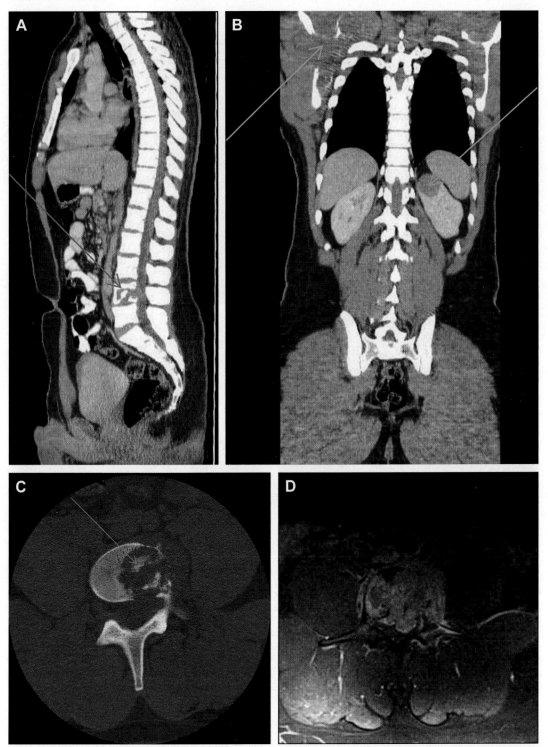

Fig. 9. A 27-year-old man with diffuse large B-cell lymphoma involving the lumbar spine. (*A*) Sagittal and (*B*) coronal reformat CT images reveal a destructive lytic lesion in the L4 vertebral body (*red arrow*), with other lesions in the right scapula and left kidney (*green arrows*). A CT-guided biopsy of the scapula lesion was performed (not shown). (*C*) Axial CT image demonstrates bony sequestrum (*blue arrow*), which can be seen with infection or lymphoma. (*D*) Axial postgadolinium MR image shows enhancing tumor, extending from the vertebral body into the epidural space. Diffuse large B-cell lymphoma is the most common high-grade or aggressive non-Hodgkin lymphoma.

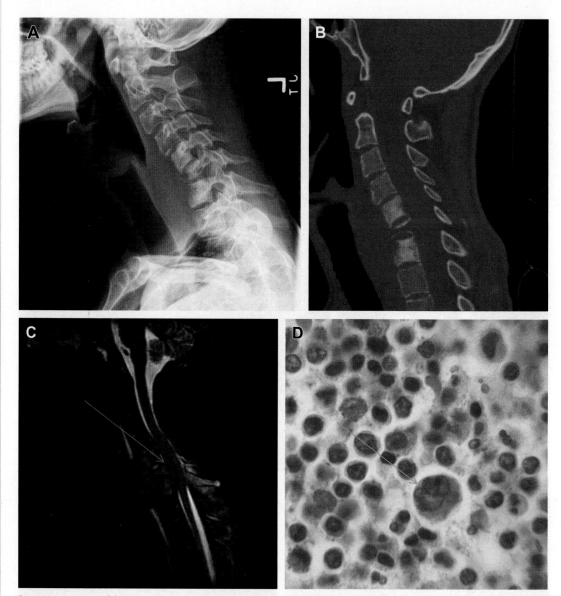

Fig. 10. A 19-year-old man with chronic intermittent neck to arm pain. (*A*, *B*) Cervical spine radiographs and subsequent CT reveal abnormal sclerosis of the C5–C7 vertebral bodies, pathologic compression of the C6 vertebral body, and widening of the prevertebral soft tissues. (*C*) Sagittal T2W image with fat saturation confirms a hypointense mass in the lower cervical vertebrae, with epidural spread into the spinal canal (*red arrow*). With elevated inflammatory markers (white blood cell/erythrocyte sedimentation rate/C-reactive protein), the preliminary diagnosis was osteomyelitis. (*D*) Histopathology (hematoxylin and eosin stain, 1000× total magnification) from open biopsy at cord decompression shows a Reed-Sternberg cell (*green arrow*), consistent with Hodgkin lymphoma (nodular sclerosing), which is more likely to cause bony sclerosis than non-Hodgkin lymphoma.

enhancement.[73,74] These findings are nonspecific and can be seen with other epidural neoplasms (eg, metastasis or leukemia) and with non-neoplastic conditions (eg, abscess or hematoma) in the appropriate clinical setting. Although hypermetabolism is also nonspecific, PET is useful for staging epidural lymphoma, often caused by FDG-avid subtypes.[75]

Similar to previous discussion with vertebral lymphoma, radiation therapy and chemotherapy are the mainstay of treatment, with surgical intervention reserved for diagnostic biopsy or spinal canal decompression. There is a trend toward combined modality therapy, which has been shown to offer a survival benefit over radiation therapy alone.[76] There is no significant difference in the 5-year survival between primary spinal epidural lymphoma and early-stage lymphoma presenting at other sites.[77] The most aggressive subtype is Burkitt lymphoma, which causes fulminant epidural lymphoma in pediatric patients, with typical survival measured in months (**Fig. 11**).[78] When comparing adult patients with spinal cord compression due to epidural tumor, the prognosis for neurologic recovery and overall survival is more favorable with earlier treatment and with lymphoma over metastatic carcinoma.[77]

LYMPHOMA OF THE INTRADURAL SPACE

In parallel with the vertebral and extradural compartments, lymphoma of the spinal cord and cauda equina is more often seen in the setting of secondary dissemination rather than as the primary site of origin. Hematogenous seeding of the leptomeninges by systemic lymphoma can manifest with abnormal enhancement on the surface of the spinal cord and nerve roots, which may then invade the neural parenchyma along perivascular spaces. Isolated lymphoma arising within the spinal cord is the least

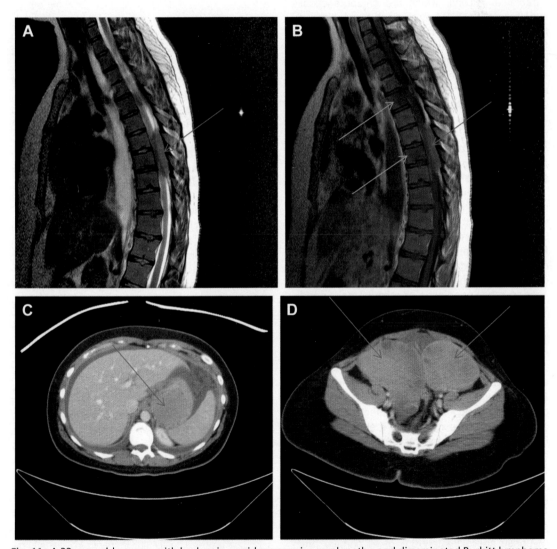

Fig. 11. A 23-year-old woman with back pain, rapid progressive myelopathy, and disseminated Burkitt lymphoma involving the thoracic spine. (*A*) Sagittal T2W and (*B*) postgadolinium images reveal a homogeneous enhancing mass in the dorsal epidural space at T7–T9 (*red arrows*) with cord compression and vertebral lesions at T5/T8 (*green arrows*). (*C*, *D*) Abdomen/pelvis CT reveals additional masses in the stomach and ovaries (*blue arrows*). Burkitt lymphoma is a rare and aggressive type of B-cell neoplasm, which more commonly affects children.

common form of primary central nervous system lymphoma, accounting for approximately 1% of cases.[8] This is primarily a disease of middle-aged and older adults, who present with nonspecific symptoms of progressive myelopathy. In a retrospective study of 14 patients identified over 14 years at the Mayo Clinic, diagnosis was delayed a median of 8 months, often mistaken for demyelinating disease.[79]

Typical CSF findings include elevated protein (without oligoclonal bands), elevated white cells, and decreased glucose. Typical MRI findings include an expansile and enhancing intramedullary lesion, isointense to spinal cord on T1W images and hyperintense on T2W images (in contrast to intracranial lesions, which are characteristically hypointense).[80] PET may be used for staging and to confirm FDG hypermetabolism. Many of these findings are nonspecific and shared with inflammatory disorders of the spinal cord, including demyelinating disease, infectious myelitis, and neurosarcoidosis. Sensitivity of CSF cytology in CNS lymphoma has been estimated to be approximately 30%, with a similar diagnostic yield for spinal cord biopsies in unexplained myelopathy.[81,82] Methotrexate is effective at penetrating the blood brain barrier and may be supplemented by other chemotherapy or radiation.

Lymphoma involvement of cranial or peripheral nerves is also known as neurolymphomatosis, which can affect the cauda equina in the lumbar spine. One literature review published in 2014 found only 15 previous case reports of primary cauda equina lymphoma.[83] The imaging finding of thickened enhancing nerve roots can also be seen in other neoplastic or inflammatory conditions, therefore CSF cytology or surgical biopsy is necessary for diagnosis. As for spinal cord lymphoma, diffuse large B-cell subtype is most commonly responsible, with histologic infiltration of the nerve tissue by CD20-positive tumor cells. Immunodeficiency is a risk factor for EBV-associated lymphoma, whereas human T-cell lymphotropic virus (HTLV) infection may predispose to the rare intradural T-cell lymphoma.[84] Prognosis is worse for intradural than vertebral or extradural lymphoma, with fewer than 50% of patients surviving 2 years after diagnosis.[79]

SUMMARY

PCNSL and its variants, once extremely rare, now comprise approximately 6% of all primary brain tumors, primarily from the strong association with immunocompromised population groups. The characteristic imaging appearance of PCNSL is one of a periventricular mass that is

> **Box 5**
> **What referring physician needs to know**
>
> - Second most common intracranial mass in an adult immunocompromised patient is PCNSL (toxoplasmosis is slightly more common overall). In the immunocompromised pediatric population, PCNSL is the most common intracranial mass.
> - Metabolic imaging (PET/SPECT) may provide more rapid distinction from toxoplasmosis.
> - Histopathologic analysis is required for diagnosis and often facilitated by stereotactic biopsy.

hyperattenuated on CT, mildly hypointense compared with surrounding vasogenic edema on T2W MR images, and nearly always shows at least some enhancement on postcontrast imaging. Basal ganglia lesions are common. The variant forms have more diverse imaging manifestations. Confirmation of diagnosis is often facilitated through stereotactic biopsy. Modern multiagent chemotherapy combined with monoclonal antibody therapy has led to remarkable progress in overall survival and remissions and ongoing therapeutic modifications remain an area of intense interest in the successful management of this aggressive disease (**Box 5**).

Extranodal lymphoma of the spine is more often caused by secondary dissemination from systemic disease and is less often the primary site of origin. Like other spinal neoplasms, primary lymphomas may be categorized by site of origin into anatomic compartments: vertebral, extradural, and intradural. Primary bone lymphoma of the vertebral column has nonspecific imaging and can be misdiagnosed as tuberculous spondylitis when B symptoms are present. Primary spinal epidural lymphoma is most common in the thoracic spine and hypothesized to arise from lymphoid tissue rests associated with the venous plexus. Primary intramedullary spinal cord lymphoma and primary cauda equina lymphoma are rare forms of primary CNS lymphoma and neurolymphomatosis, respectively.

REFERENCES

1. Batchelor T, Loeffler JS. Primary CNS lymphoma. J Clin Oncol 2006;24(8):1281–8.

2. Deckert M, Paulus W. Malignant lymphomas. In: Louis DN, Ohgaki H, Wiestler OD, et al, editors. WHO classification of tumours of the central

nervous system. 4th edition. Lyon: IARC Press; 2007. p. 188–92.

3. Kadan-Lottick NS, Skluzacek MC, Gurney JG. Decreasing incidence rates of primary central nervous system lymphoma. Cancer 2002;95(1): 193–202.

4. Bataille B, Delwail V, Menet E, et al. Primary intracerebral malignant lymphoma: report of 248 cases. J Neurosurg 2000;92(2):261–6.

5. Kuker W, Nagele T, Korfel A, et al. Primary central nervous system lymphomas (PCNSL): MRI features at presentation in 100 patients. J Neurooncol 2005; 72(2):169–77.

6. Ferreri AJ, Blay JY, Reni M, et al. Prognostic scoring system for primary CNS lymphomas: the International Extranodal Lymphoma Study Group experience. J Clin Oncol 2003; 21(2):266–72.

7. Louveau A, Smirnov I, Keyes TJ, et al. Structural and functional features of central nervous system lymphatic vessels. Nature 2015;523(7560):337–41.

8. Koeller KK, Smirniotopoulos JG, Jones RV. Primary central nervous system lymphoma: radiologic-pathologic correlation. Radiographics 1997;17(6): 1497–526.

9. Choi JS, Nam DH, Ko YH, et al. Primary central nervous system lymphoma in Korea: comparison of B- and T-cell lymphomas. Am J Surg Pathol 2003; 27(7):919–28.

10. Hayakawa T, Takakura K, Abe H, et al. Primary central nervous system lymphoma in Japan–a retrospective, co-operative study by CNS-Lymphoma Study Group in Japan. J Neurooncol 1994;19(3): 197–215.

11. Herrlinger U, Klingel K, Meyermann R, et al. Central nervous system Hodgkin's lymphoma without systemic manifestation: case report and review of the literature. Acta Neuropathol 2000;99(6): 709–14.

12. Ferracini R, Bergmann M, Pileri S, et al. Primary T-cell lymphoma of the central nervous system. Clin Neuropathol 1995;14(3):125–9.

13. Villegas E, Villa S, Lopez-Guillermo A, et al. Primary central nervous system lymphoma of T-cell origin: description of two cases and review of the literature. J Neurooncol 1997;34(2): 157–61.

14. Alderson L, Fetell MR, Sisti M, et al. Sentinel lesions of primary CNS lymphoma. J Neurol Neurosurg Psychiatry 1996;60(1):102–5.

15. Weingarten KL, Zimmerman RD, Leeds NE. Spontaneous regression of intracerebral lymphoma. Radiology 1983;149(3):721–4.

16. Haldorsen IS, Espeland A, Larsson EM. Central nervous system lymphoma: characteristic findings on traditional and advanced imaging. AJNR Am J Neuroradiol 2011;32(6):984–92.

17. Bellinzona M, Roser F, Ostertag H, et al. Surgical removal of primary central nervous system lymphomas (PCNSL) presenting as space occupying lesions: a series of 33 cases. Eur J Surg Oncol 2005;31(1):100–5.

18. DeAngelis LM, Yahalom J, Heinemann MH, et al. Primary CNS lymphoma: combined treatment with chemotherapy and radiotherapy. Neurology 1990; 40(1):80–6.

19. Pels H, Schmidt-Wolf IG, Glasmacher A, et al. Primary central nervous system lymphoma: results of a pilot and phase II study of systemic and intraventricular chemotherapy with deferred radiotherapy. J Clin Oncol 2003;21(24): 4489–95.

20. Illerhaus G, Marks R, Ihorst G, et al. High-dose chemotherapy with autologous stem-cell transplantation and hyperfractionated radiotherapy as first-line treatment of primary CNS lymphoma. J Clin Oncol 2006;24(24):3865–70.

21. Abrey LE, Moskowitz CH, Mason WP, et al. Intensive methotrexate and cytarabine followed by high-dose chemotherapy with autologous stem-cell rescue in patients with newly diagnosed primary CNS lymphoma: an intent-to-treat analysis. J Clin Oncol 2003;21(22):4151–6.

22. Madle M, Kramer I, Lehners N, et al. The influence of rituximab, high-dose therapy followed by autologous stem cell transplantation, and age in patients with primary CNS lymphoma. Ann Hematol 2015;94(11): 1853–7.

23. Holubar K. The man behind the eponym. Angioendotheliomatosis proliferans systemisata (Tappeiner-Pfleger disease). A short description of the disease and biographical notes on the eponyms. Am J Dermatopathol 1984;6(6):537–9.

24. Pfleger L, Tappeiner J. Zur Kenntnis der systemisierten Endotheliomatose der cutanen Blutgefasse. Hautarzt 1959;10:259–63.

25. Tappeiner J, Pfleger L. Angioendotheliomatosis proliferans systematisata. A clinically and pathohistologically new disease picture. Hautarzt 1963;14: 67–70 [in German].

26. Orwat DE, Batalis NI. Intravascular large B-cell lymphoma. Arch Pathol Lab Med 2012;136(3): 333–8.

27. Ferreri AJ, Campo E, Seymour JF, et al. Intravascular lymphoma: clinical presentation, natural history, management and prognostic factors in a series of 38 cases, with special emphasis on the 'cutaneous variant'. Br J Haematol 2004;127(2): 173–83.

28. Williams RL, Meltzer CC, Smirniotopoulos JG, et al. Cerebral MR imaging in intravascular lymphomatosis. AJNR Am J Neuroradiol 1998;19(3):427–31.

29. Baehring JM, Henchcliffe C, Ledezma CJ, et al. Intravascular lymphoma: magnetic resonance

imaging correlates of disease dynamics within the central nervous system. J Neurol Neurosurg Psychiatry 2005;76(4):540–4.

30. Imai H, Kajimoto K, Taniwaki M, et al. Intravascular large B-cell lymphoma presenting with mass lesions in the central nervous system: a report of five cases. Pathol Int 2004;54(4):231–6.

31. Kenez J, Barsi P, Majtenyi K, et al. Can intravascular lymphomatosis mimic sinus thrombosis? A case report with 8 months' follow-up and fatal outcome. Neuroradiology 2000;42(6):436–40.

32. Ponzoni M, Ferreri AJ. Intravascular lymphoma: a neoplasm of 'homeless' lymphocytes? Hematol Oncol 2006;24(3):105–12.

33. Keswani A, Bigio E, Grimm S. Lymphomatosis cerebri presenting with orthostatic hypotension, anorexia, and paraparesis. J Neurooncol 2012; 109(3):581–6.

34. Kitai R, Hashimoto N, Yamate K, et al. Lymphomatosis cerebri: clinical characteristics, neuroimaging, and pathological findings. Brain Tumor Pathol 2012;29(1):47–53.

35. Pandit L, Chickabasaviah Y, Raghothaman A, et al. Lymphomatosis cerebri–a rare cause of leukoencephalopathy. J Neurol Sci 2010;293(1–2):122–4.

36. Rollins KE, Kleinschmidt-DeMasters BK, Corboy JR, et al. Lymphomatosis cerebri as a cause of white matter dementia. Hum Pathol 2005;36(3):282–90.

37. Dunleavy K, Roschewski M, Wilson WH. Lymphomatoid granulomatosis and other Epstein-Barr virus associated lymphoproliferative processes. Curr Hematol Malig Rep 2012;7(3):208–15.

38. Liu H, Chen J, Yu D, et al. Lymphomatoid granulomatosis involving the central nervous system: a case report and review of the literature. Oncol Lett 2014;7(6):1843–6.

39. Patsalides AD, Atac G, Hedge U, et al. Lymphomatoid granulomatosis: abnormalities of the brain at MR imaging. Radiology 2005;237(1): 265–73.

40. Kapila A, Gupta KL, Garcia JH. CT and MR of lymphomatoid granulomatosis of the CNS: report of four cases and review of the literature. AJNR Am J Neuroradiol 1988;9(6):1139–43.

41. Cavaliere R, Petroni G, Lopes MB, et al, International Primary Central Nervous System Lymphoma Collaborative Group. Primary central nervous system post-transplantation lymphoproliferative disorder: an International Primary Central Nervous System Lymphoma Collaborative Group Report. Cancer 2010;116(4):863–70.

42. Castellano-Sanchez AA, Li S, Qian J, et al. Primary central nervous system posttransplant lymphoproliferative disorders. Am J Clin Pathol 2004;121(2):246–53.

43. Harris NL, Jaffe ES, Diebold J, et al. World Health Organization classification of neoplastic diseases of the hematopoietic and lymphoid tissues: report of the Clinical Advisory Committee meeting-Airlie House, Virginia, November 1997. J Clin Oncol 1999;17(12):3835–49.

44. Buell JF, Gross TG, Hanaway MJ, et al. Posttransplant lymphoproliferative disorder: significance of central nervous system involvement. Transplant Proc 2005;37(2):954–5.

45. Pickhardt PJ, Wippold FJ 2nd. Neuroimaging in posttransplantation lymphoproliferative disorder. AJR Am J Roentgenol 1999;172(4):1117–21.

46. Korner S, Raab P, Brandis A, et al. Spontaneous regression of an intracerebral lymphoma (ghost tumor) in a liver-engrafted patient. Neurologist 2011; 17(4):218–21.

47. Arita H, Izumoto S, Kinoshita M, et al. Posttransplant lymphoproliferative disorders of the central nervous system after kidney transplantation: single center experience over 40 years. Two case reports. Neurol Med Chir (Tokyo) 2010;50(12):1079–83.

48. Haque S, Law M, Abrey LE, et al. Imaging of lymphoma of the central nervous system, spine, and orbit. Radiol Clin North Am 2008;46(2):339–61.

49. Mikhaeel NG. Primary bone lymphoma. Clin Oncol 2012;24(5):366–70.

50. Ramadan KM, Shenkier T, Sehn LH, et al. A clinicopathological retrospective study of 131 patients with primary bone lymphoma: a population-based study of successively treated cohorts from the British Columbia Cancer Agency. Ann Oncol 2007;18(1):129–35.

51. Chang CM, Chen HC, Yang Y, et al. Surgical decompression improves recovery from neurological deficit and may provide a survival benefit in patients with diffuse large B-cell lymphoma-associated spinal cord compression: a case-series study. World J Surg Oncol 2013;11:90.

52. Peng X, Wan Y, Chen Y, et al. Primary non-Hodgkin's lymphoma of the spine with neurologic compression treated by radiotherapy and chemotherapy alone or combined with surgical decompression. Oncol Rep 2009;21(5):1269–75.

53. Mulligan ME, McRae GA, Murphey MD. Imaging features of primary lymphoma of bone. AJR Am J Roentgenol 1999;173(6):1691–7.

54. Krishnan A, Shirkhoda A, Tehranzadeh J, et al. Primary bone lymphoma: radiographic-MR imaging correlation. Radiographics 2003;23(6):1371–83.

55. Abdel Razek AA, Castillo M. Imaging appearance of primary bony tumors and pseudo-tumors of the spine. J Neuroradiol 2010;37(1):37–50.

56. Mulligan ME, Kransdorf MJ. Sequestra in primary lymphoma of bone: prevalence and radiologic features. AJR Am J Roentgenol 1993;160(6):1245–8.

57. Abdelwahab IF, Miller TT, Hermann G, et al. Transarticular invasion of joints by bone tumors: hypothesis. Skeletal Radiol 1991;20(4):279–83.

58. Huang B, Li CQ, Liu T, et al. Primary non-Hodgkin's lymphoma of the lumbar vertebrae mimicking tuberculous spondylitis: a case report. Arch Orthop Trauma Surg 2009;129(12):1621–5.

59. Adegboye OA. Non-Hodgkin's lymphoma "masquerading" as Pott's disease in a 13-year old boy. Indian J Med Paediatr Oncol 2011;32(2):101–4.

60. Uehara M, Takahashi J, Hirabayashi H, et al. Hodgkin's disease of the thoracic vertebrae. Spine J 2013;13(8):e59–63.

61. Graham TS. The ivory vertebra sign. Radiology 2005;235(2):614–5.

62. Stiglbauer R, Augustin I, Kramer J, et al. MRI in the diagnosis of primary lymphoma of bone: correlation with histopathology. J Comput Assist Tomogr 1992; 16(2):248–53.

63. Hicks DG, Gokan T, O'Keefe RJ, et al. Primary lymphoma of bone. Correlation of magnetic resonance imaging features with cytokine production by tumor cells. Cancer 1995;75(4):973–80.

64. Moog F, Kotzerke J, Reske SN. FDG PET can replace bone scintigraphy in primary staging of malignant lymphoma. J Nucl Med 1999;40(9): 1407–13.

65. Paes FM, Kalkanis DG, Sideras PA, et al. FDG PET/CT of extranodal involvement in non-Hodgkin lymphoma and Hodgkin disease. Radiographics 2010; 30(1):269–91.

66. Cugati G, Singh M, Pande A, et al. Primary spinal epidural lymphomas. J Craniovertebr Junction Spine 2011;2(1):3–11.

67. Cağavi F, Kalayci M, Tekin IO, et al. Primary spinal extranodal Hodgkin's disease at two levels. Clin Neurol Neurosurg 2006;108(2):168–73.

68. Barnard M, Perez-Ordoñez B, Rowed DW, et al. Primary spinal epidural mantle cell lymphoma: case report. Neurosurgery 2000;47(5):1239–41.

69. Monnard V, Sun A, Epelbaum R, et al. Primary spinal epidural lymphoma: patients' profile, outcome, and prognostic factors: a multicenter Rare Cancer Network study. Int J Radiat Oncol Biol Phys 2006; 65(3):817–23.

70. Raco A, Cervoni L, Salvati M, et al. Primary spinal epidural non-Hodgkin's lymphomas in childhood: a review of 6 cases. Acta Neurochir (Wien) 1997; 139(6):526–8.

71. Epelbaum R, Haim N, Ben-Shahar M, et al. Non-Hodgkin's lymphoma presenting with spinal epidural involvement. Cancer 1986;58(9):2120–4.

72. Mora J, Wollner N. Primary epidural non-Hodgkin lymphoma: spinal cord compression syndrome as the initial form of presentation in childhood non-Hodgkin lymphoma. Med Pediatr Oncol 1999; 32(2):102–5.

73. Boukobza M, Mazel C, Touboul E. Primary vertebral and spinal epidural non-Hodgkin's lymphoma with spinal cord compression. Neuroradiology 1996; 38(4):333–7.

74. Mascalchi M, Torselli P, Falaschi F, et al. MRI of spinal epidural lymphoma. Neuroradiology 1995;37(4): 303–7.

75. Ho L, Valenzuela D, Negahban A, et al. Primary spinal epidural non-Hodgkin lymphoma demonstrated by FDG PET/CT. Clin Nucl Med 2010;35(7):487–9.

76. Rathmell AJ, Gospodarowicz MK, Sutcliffe SB, et al. Localized extradural lymphoma: survival, relapse pattern and functional outcome. The Princess Margaret Hospital Lymphoma Group. Radiother Oncol 1992;24(1):14–20.

77. Haddad P, Thaell JF, Kiely JM, et al. Lymphoma of the spinal extradural space. Cancer 1976;38(4): 1862–6.

78. Mizugami T, Mikata A, Hajikano H, et al. Primary spinal epidural Burkitt's lymphoma. Surg Neurol 1987; 28(2):158–62.

79. Flanagan EP, O'Neill BP, Porter AB, et al. Primary intramedullary spinal cord lymphoma. Neurology 2011;77(8):784–91.

80. Koeller KK, Rosenblum RS, Morrison AL. Neoplasms of the spinal cord and filum terminale: radiologic-pathologic correlation. Radiographics 2000;20(6): 1721–49.

81. Fitzsimmons A, Upchurch K, Batchelor T. Clinical features and diagnosis of primary central nervous system lymphoma. Hematol Oncol Clin North Am 2005;19(4):689–703.

82. Cohen-Gadol AA, Zikel OM, Miller GM, et al. Spinal cord biopsy: a review of 38 cases. Neurosurgery 2003;52(4):806–15.

83. Nakashima H, Imagama S, Ito Z, et al. Primary cauda equina lymphoma: case report and literature review. Nagoya J Med Sci 2014;76(3–4):349–54.

84. Urasaki E, Yamada H, Tokimura T, et al. T-cell type primary spinal intramedullary lymphoma associated with human T-cell lymphotropic virus type I after a renal transplant: case report. Neurosurgery 1996; 38(5):1036–9.

Primary Extranodal Lymphoma of the Thorax

Seth J. Kligerman, MD[a,b,*], Teri J. Franks, MD[c], Jeffrey R. Galvin, MD[a,b,d]

KEYWORDS

• Lymphoma • Thorax • Extranodal • Primary • MALT • Thymus • Pleura

KEY POINTS

- Primary pulmonary lymphomas (PPLs) represent a pathologically heterogeneous group of disorders that often share imaging features, which include peribronchovascular nodules and masses or areas of nonresolving consolidation.
- Primary mediastinal B-cell lymphoma is an extranodal non-Hodgkin lymphoma (NHL) seen in younger patients that has imaging and pathologic features that demonstrate some degree of overlap with Hodgkin lymphoma (HL).
- Primary lymphomas of the pleural space are rare and associated with concomitant viral infections.

INTRODUCTION

Neoplasms originating in lymphoid tissue are common, 2015, it is estimated that there will be approximately 72,000 newly diagnosed cases of non-Hodgkin lymphoma (NHL) and 9000 newly diagnosed cases of hodgkin lymphomas (HLs) in the United States.[1] A vast majority of these cases represent systemic diseases that arise from and spread to lymphoid tissue throughout the body and most commonly involve lymph nodes, bone marrow, and spleen. Lymphoid tissue exists, however, in numerous places throughout the body and, therefore, malignant and nonmalignant lymphoid proliferations can be seen in and isolated to various organs and tissues. Although uncommon, these primary extranodal lymphomas occur throughout the thorax and can involve the lung, mediastinum, and pleura.

PRIMARY PULMONARY EXTRANODAL NEOPLASTIC LYMPHOID PROLIFERATIONS

Lymphomatous lesions of the lung can occur through 3 mechanisms. In most instances, either HL or NHL seeds the lung through hematogenous dissemination or directly invades the pulmonary parenchyma via extension from adjacent hilar or mediastinal lymph nodes. These secondary malignant manifestations are more common than primary pulmonary lymphoproliferative disorders because secondary pulmonary involvement can occur in up to 24% of patients with NHL and up to 38% of patients with HL.[2] The third mechanism, which is the least common, occurs when there is a primary clonal lymphoid proliferation that originates in the lung.[3] These primary pulmonary lymphoproliferative disorders are rare and represent only 0.3% of all primary pulmonary malignancies,

Disclaimer for T.J. Franks: The views expressed in this article are those of the author and do not reflect the official policy of the Department of Defense or the United States Government.

[a] Chest Imaging, Department of Radiology and Nuclear Medicine, University of Maryland School of Medicine, 22 South Greene Street, Baltimore, MD 21201, USA; [b] Chest Imaging, American Institute for Radiologic Pathology, 1010 Wayne Ave, Suite 320, Silver Spring, MD 2091, USA; [c] Pulmonary and Mediastinal Pathology, Department of Defense, Joint Pathology Center, 606 Stephen Sitter Ave, Silver Spring, MD 20910-1290, USA; [d] Pulmonary and Critical Care Medicine, Department of Internal Medicine, University of Maryland School of Medicine, 22 South Greene Street, Baltimore, MD 21201, USA

* Corresponding author. Department of Radiology and Nuclear Medicine, University of Maryland School of Medicine, 22 South Greene Street, Baltimore, MD 21201.
E-mail address: skligerman@umm.edu

less than 1% of all NHL cases and only 3% to 4% of all extranodal manifestation of NHL.[4]

Primary pulmonary lymphomas (PPLs) represents a monoclonal proliferation of lymphoid tissue in the lungs in patients with no detectable extrathoracic lymphoma for at least 3 months after initial diagnosis.[2] These lesions arise from bronchus-associated lymphoid tissue (BALT), which is 1 component of the complex pulmonary lymphatic system. BALT is a specific type of mucosa-associated lymphoid tissue (MALT) in the lungs that is involved with the body's immune response to inhaled antigens. BALT represents an organized cluster of central B cells surrounded by a peripheral rim of T cells and lacks germinal centers when antigenic stimulation is absent. Although afferent lymph channels are absent, BALT drains to regional lymph nodes via efferent lymphatic channels.

Although absent at birth, BALT begins to develop in infants and young children due to antigenic stimulation. Although this tissue regresses in healthy adults, it reappears in those who undergo acute or chronic antigenic stimulation and can be seen in adults with acute or chronic infection, chronic bronchial inflammation (asthma), collagen vascular diseases, or AIDS and in cigarette smokers (Fig. 1).[5,6] It is the chronic antigenic stimulation of BALT that leads to a variety of benign and malignant lymphoid lesions that are visualized on imaging. In some instances, chronic stimulation

of BALT can lead to various types of lymphoid lesions, such as follicular bronchiolitis, lymphocytic interstitial pneumonia, and MALT lymphoma, arising in a single patient.[6–9]

The most common type is the more indolent low-grade marginal zone B-cell lymphoma of MALT lymphoma, which represents between 60% and 80% of cases of PPL.[10,11] The more aggressive diffuse large B-cell lymphomas (DLBCLs) represent approximately 10% to 25% of cases and are the second most common form of PPL.[6,12] Other rarer causes of PPL include follicular lymphoma, Burkitt lymphoma, and T-cell lymphoma. Primary pulmonary HL PPHL is extremely rare and usually arises from direct extension of mediastinal disease or is associated with disseminated disease. Fewer than 70 cases of PPHL have been reported in the literature since 1927.[13] Lymphomatoid granulomatosis (LG) is a rare form of PPL with a poor overall survival. Although it is generally accepted as a lymphoproliferative disorder, controversy exists in regards to its diagnosis, taxonomy, and relationship to other forms of PPL.[14]

MUCOSA-ASSOCIATED LYMPHOID TISSUE LYMPHOMA (LOW-GRADE MARGINAL ZONE B-CELL LYMPHOMA OF MUCOSA-ASSOCIATED LYMPHOID TISSUE)

As discussed previously, MALT lymphoma is the most common PPL to involve the lung. Most patients are in their sixth to seventh decades of life and slightly more than half of patients are women.[11,15] At the time of diagnosis, approximately half of the patients are asymptomatic. When symptoms are present, they are usually nonspecific and include cough, mild dyspnea, chest pain, and hemoptysis. Extrapulmonary manifestations, which are restricted to general signs, such as fever and weight loss, given the definition of PPL, occur in less than one-quarter of patients.[3]

A majority of patients have some form of chronic antigenic stimulation, which is associated with growth of BALT.[16] In 1 large meta-analysis, 45% of patients had a history of smoking, 9% of patients had a history of exposure to toxic substances, and 19% had a known preexisting lung disease.[15] Collagen vascular diseases are seen in approximately 10% to 29% of patients with MALT lymphoma, a majority of which have Sjögren syndrome.[17–19] Although usually associated with the development of more aggressive lymphomas, MALT lymphoma can also be seen in patients with systemic lupus or patients with rheumatoid arthritis (RA), particularly in those with RA treated

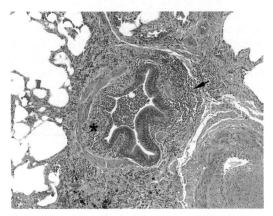

Fig. 1. Smoking-related BALT hyperplasia. Medium-power microscopic image (original magnification, ×100; hematoxylin-eosin stain) demonstrates a small airway with submucosal and adventitial lymphoid infiltrates (*arrow*) typical of BALT hyperplasia. This is associated with smoking-related small airway injury, including respiratory bronchiolitis, characterized by luminal accumulation of yellow-brown pigmented macrophages; submucosal organization; and chronic inflammation (*asterisk*).

with methotrexate.[20,21] Chronic infections, such as HIV and hepatitis C, also are common.[16,22]

The imaging of MALT lymphoma varies significantly. Although solitary lesions occur, most patients have multiple lesions (**Fig. 2**), which can be unilateral or bilateral.[6,23–26] These lesions can have a variety of configurations ranging from well-defined to poorly defined nodules or masses, which often have a peribronchovascular distribution. In other instances, lesions can appear as areas of consolidation, which are often described as masslike or nodular in appearance (**Fig. 3**) Attenuation can also vary with lesions appearing solid, mixed solid and ground glass, or pure ground glass in attenuation. Most lesions measure less than 5 cm in diameter and air bronchograms or areas of bronchiectasis within the larger lesions are often present. Consolidation of an entire lobe can, however, occur (**Fig. 4**). In a majority of patients, follow-up CT imaging shows no appreciable growth in lesions, which can be stable for many years.[23] This stability excludes many acute causes of consolidation. A similar pattern on CT can be seen, however, in other entities, such as organizing pneumonia, eosinophilic pneumonia, alveolar pattern of sarcoidosis, multifocal adenocarcinoma/adenocarcinoma in situ, and other benign lymphoproliferative diseases, such as nodular lymphoid hyperplasia and lymphoid interstitial pneumonia (LIP).

Macroscopically, MALT lymphoma typically shows cream-colored consolidation of the lung parenchyma (**Fig. 5**). Microscopically, MALT lymphoma is comprised of sheets of monoclonal lymphocytes with interspersed plasma cells (**Fig. 6**). A lymphangitic pattern of infiltration

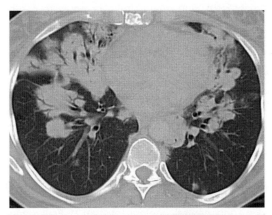

Fig. 2. Primary MALT lymphoma of the lung. Axial CT image acquired through the lower lung zones in a 60-year-old woman who presents with dyspnea demonstrates multiple masslike nodules that follow the bronchovascular bundles. There are numerous air bronchograms with normal airway architecture.

coalescing to form destructive masses that efface the lung parenchyma is also a common architectural pattern.[27] This, in conjunction with extension of B cells beyond the confines of reactive lymphoid follicles, helps to differentiate MALT lymphoma from benign lymphoid lesions, such as follicular bronchiolitis, LIP, and nodular lymphoid hyperplasia.[28] Lymphoepithelial lesions, representing areas of invasion of the bronchial epithelium by lymphoid cells, are present but can be seen in both malignant and benign lymphoid proliferations. Although LIP and primary MALT lymphoma of the lung can coexist in the same patient, it is unlikely that there is transformation of LIP into a malignant process (**Fig. 7**).[2] Amyloid deposition can also be seen in conjunction with MALT lymphoma as well as in patients with benign pulmonary lymphocytic infiltration.[29–31] Survival in patients with pulmonary MALT lymphoma is overall favorable. There is a 5-year survival rate of greater than 80% and a median survival greater than 10 years.[3]

DIFFUSE LARGE B-CELL LYMPHOMA

DLBCL most commonly is a system disease. Although less common than primary pulmonary MALT lymphoma, 10% to 19% of cases of PPL are secondary to DLBCL.[7,12] Although DLBCL can occur via a primary proliferation, it can also arise from the transformation of the more indolent MALT lymphoma into a more aggressive DLBCL.[6,19,32] Many patients who develop high-grade PPL have some underlying chronic infectious or inflammatory process, such as HIV infection, chronic immunosuppression, or a collagen vascular disease.[3,33]

Microscopically, sheets of atypical lymphocytes form solid lesions that replace the underlying architecture of the lung (**Fig. 8**).[13] Although necrosis and cavitation are common, normal and diseased lung are usually sharply demarcated. On imaging, the features of MALT lymphoma and primary DLBCL can overlap. In both cases, patients can present with solitary or multiple nodules or areas of consolidation. Cavitation and/or necrosis is a common feature with DLBCL and is more frequent than in cases of MALT lymphoma (**Fig. 9**).[16] Although long-term survival in patients with primary pulmonary DLBCL has historically been poor, a recent study demonstrated a 10-year event-free survival of 90%.[3,34]

LYMPHOMATOID GRANULOMATOSIS

Microscopically, LG is an angiocentric (**Fig. 10**) and angiodestructive (**Fig. 11**) process characterized by

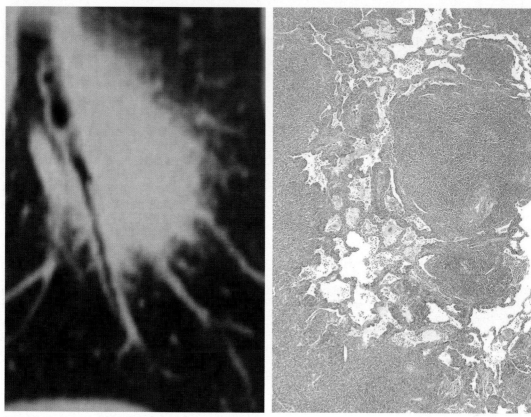

Fig. 3. Primary MALT lymphoma of the lung. Coronal reconstruction of axial CT data (*left*) in a 64-year-old white woman with incidentally discovered masslike consolidation in the left lower lobe. Typical findings include an air bronchogram and an indistinct border with multiple surrounding micronodules. Correlative histology (*right*) (H&E, 20×) from the periphery of the mass demonstrates variable, lymphocytic infiltration of the alveolar walls, resulting in an indistinct nodular margin on imaging.

the presence of small numbers of Epstein-Barr virus (EBV)-positive B cells surrounded by a more prominent inflammatory background composed of polyclonal T cells, plasma cells, and histiocytes.[35] Although speculated to have a viral pathogenesis when first described by Leibow in the 1970s,[36] the association with a virus was not proved until 1990 when Katzenstein and Peiper[37] identified EBV DNA in 72% of cases. The EBV-positive B cells are large in size, demonstrate some degree of atypia, express CD20, and are negative for CD15. The presence of these B cells is a key feature in LG and the number of these cells has a linear association with survival.[14] Based on this, the World Health Organization (WHO) currently recommends that the number of these large B cells, the number that are identified as EBV positive by in situ hybridization, and the degree of necrosis be used to stage the disease.[14,38] In grade 1 lesions, the least common lesions, large B cells are absent or rare and fewer than 5 of these cells are EBV positive per high-power field. The B-cell

proliferation is polyclonal and necrosis is absent. In grade 2 lesions, occasional large lymphoid cells are present, and greater than or equal to 5 but fewer than or equal to 50 of these cells are EBV positive. The B-cell proliferation is oligoclonal or monoclonal and necrosis is present. In grade 3 lesions, large B cells are abundant and greater than 50 EBV-positive large B cells are seen in a single high-power field. The B-cell proliferation is monoclonal and necrosis is usually extensive. Grading of lesions is best done with surgical biopsy because bronchoscopic or transthoracic biopsy can lead to undergrading.

LG affects middle-aged adults and a majority of patients are men. Although LG can occur in any part of the body, it is most common in the lung, skin, and central nervous system.[14] Fever and cough are the most common symptoms. LG can occur in isolation but some patients have a history of underlying hematopoetic disease, including lymphoma and leukemia.[39] In addition, LG can occur in patients with a congenital or acquired

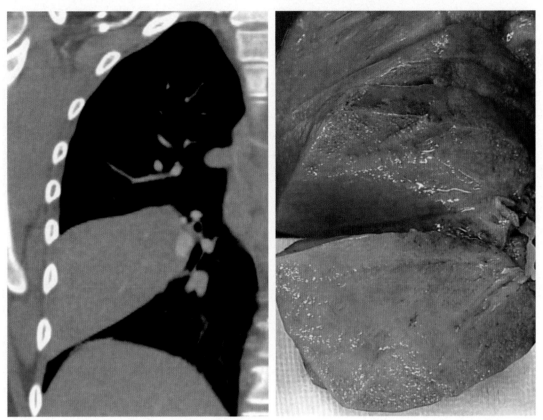

Fig. 4. Primary MALT lymphoma of the lung. Coronal reconstruction of axial CT data (*left*) in a 51-year-old woman who presents with cough. There is uniform consolidation of the middle lobe. Gross (*right*) demonstrates complete replacement of the middle lobe by lymphoma.

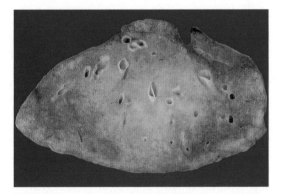

Fig. 5. Primary MALT lymphoma of lung. Gross image of lung demonstrates ill-defined cream-colored consolidation of the parenchyma typical of lymphoma. Centrally, the neoplasm effaces the architecture of alveolar walls and alveolar spaces while leaving bronchovascular bundles intact. The ill-defined border represents variable involvement of lymphatics, alveolar walls, and alveolar spaces by neoplasm.

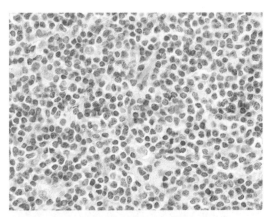

Fig. 6. Primary MALT lymphoma of lung. High-power microscopic image (original magnification, ×600; hematoxylin-eosin stain) of lung demonstrates a predominance of small to medium-sized lymphocytes admixed with fewer numbers of large lymphocytes and scattered cells with plasmacytic differentiation typical of MALT lymphoma.

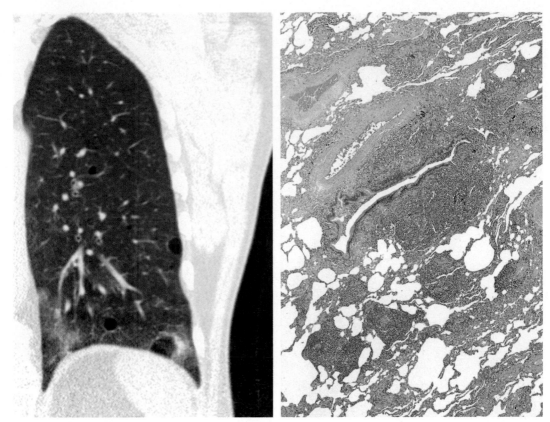

Fig. 7. Combined LIP and MALT Lymphoma. Coronal reconstruction of axial CT data (*left*) in a 62-year-old man with typical changes of lymphocytic interstitial pneumonia including thin-walled cysts in the midlung and lower lung zones along with patchy areas of ground glass and consolidation. Correlative histology (*right*) (H&E, 20×) demonstrates a combination of airway narrowing and alveolar wall widening due to infiltration with inflammatory cells. Immunohistochemistry confirms a diagnosis of primary MALT lymphoma of the lung.

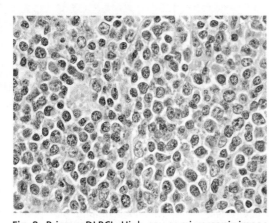

Fig. 8. Primary DLBCL. High-power microscopic image (original magnification, ×600; hematoxylin-eosin stain) of lung demonstrates large lymphoid cells with vesicular (open) nuclear chromatin and several small nucleoli typical of DLBCL with centroblastic morphology.

immunodeficiency disease and has been reported in patients with Sjögren syndrome, sarcoidosis, ulcerative colitis, primary biliary cirrhosis, retroperitoneal fibrosis, psoriasis and in those with rheumatoid arthritis treated with methotrexate.[39,40]

On radiographs, the most common finding in LG is the presence of bilateral nodules and masses[41] (**Fig. 12**). On CT, patients present with both poorly defined and well-defined peribronchovascular and septal nodules, masses, and areas of consolidation, which may have internal air bronchograms. The number of lesions varies significantly (range from 5 to 60) and although most measure less than 1 cm in diameter, masses up to 6.5 cm have been described (**Fig. 13**).[42] Fluorodeoxyglucose F 18 (FDG)–PET images show avid uptake in the lesions. These nodules can coalesce and cavitation can be seen in up to 30% of cases[43] (**Fig. 14**). Less commonly, patients can

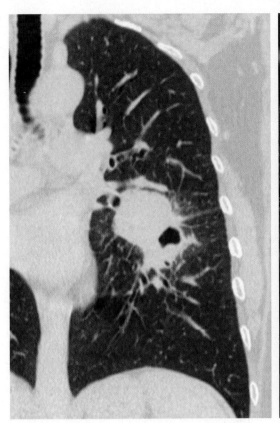
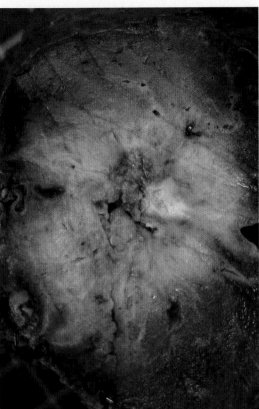

Fig. 9. DLBCL. Coronal reconstruction of axial CT data (*left*) in a 62-year-old woman with fever and malaise. The CT demonstrates a well-circumscribed mass with cavitation. The corresponding gross (*right*) demonstrates central necrosis.

present with a pattern of numerous small peribronchovascular nodules, reticulation, and architectural distortion.[42] Lymph node enlargement and effusions also are seen.[16,24]

Both prognosis and treatment are variable and depend on the grade of the lesion with both grades 2 and 3 having a poorer prognosis. Even though grade 1 lesions lack morphologic

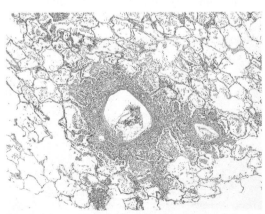

Fig. 10. LG. Low-power microscopic image (original magnification, ×40; hematoxylin-eosin stain) of lung demonstrates an angiocentric growth pattern of atypical lymphocytes and inflammatory cells typical of LG.

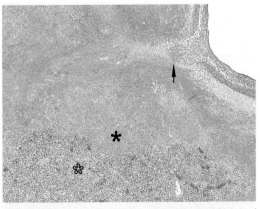

Fig. 11. LG. Low-power microscopic image (original magnification, ×40; hematoxylin-eosin stain) demonstrates lung parenchyma with dense lymphoid infiltrates (*clear asterisk*) and infarct-like tissue necrosis (*black asterisk*) due to vascular compromise (*arrow*) of a small pulmonary artery typical of the angiodestructive growth pattern of LG.

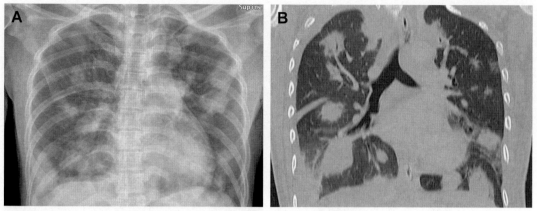

Fig. 12. LG. (*A*) Anteroposterior portable supine radiograph and (*B*) coronal reconstruction of axial CT data in a 33-year-old man with history of HIV infection demonstrate nodules of varying size involving all 5 lobes. The CT demonstrates both well-circumscribed and indistinct nodules. There is an air bronchogram in the right upper lobe nodule.

features of lymphoma, prognosis is still poor, which may be due to progression to a higher grade, biopsy variation, or the fact that pulmonary lesions can demonstrate variable grades in the same patient. In addition, patients with higher-grade disease can develop an aggressive DLBCL involving lymph nodes and the lymphoreticular system. Newer studies performed at the National Cancer Institute, however, have demonstrated improved survival.[33]

POST-TRANSPLANT LYMPHOPROLIFERATIVE DISORDER

After solid organ or bone marrow transplantation, patients can develop a range of lymphoid abnormalities, predominantly involving B cells, which can range from benign polyclonal lymphoid hyperplasia to aggressive monoclonal lymphomas.

Similar to other lymphoid proliferations, post-transplant lymphoproliferative disorder (PTLD) is associated with an EBV viral infection.[44] Although the term PTLD classically encompasses the full gambit of EBV-related lymphoproliferative states in the post-transplant patient, in most instances the term is used to denote disease states on the malignant end of the spectrum.[45]

The incidence of PTLD varies depending of the type of allograft and other coexistent risk factors. PTLD is most common after solid organ transplant, with a reported incidence from 5% to 20% in patients with lung or bowel transplant and a lower incidence of 2% to 3% in adult patients post–renal or hepatic transplantation.[46] Additional risk factors for developing PTLD in patients with solid organ transplant include a patient being EBV negative pretransplantation with subsequent infection, co-infection with cytomegalovirus, and high doses of

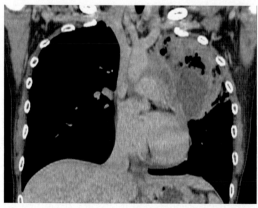

Fig. 13. LG. Coronal reconstruction of axial CT data in a 31-year-old woman with left chest pain demonstrates a large necrotic mass in the left upper lobe.

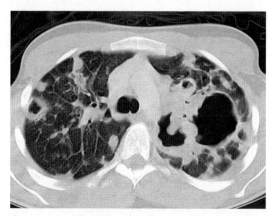

Fig. 14. LG with solid and cavitary nodules. Axial CT of the chest through the upper lung zones demonstrates both solid and cavitary nodules of varying size.

antilymphocyte antibodies for immunosuppression.[44,47] Younger age of transplantation is also associated with a 4 to 8 times risk of developing PTLD.[48]

PTLD can also occur in patients after hematopoetic stem cell transplantation although the incidence is much lower, at approximately 1%.[32,49] Additional risk factors in patients post–hematopoetic stem cell transplantation are different from those with solid organ transplantation and include T-cell–depleted donor cells, HLA-mismatched transplant, immunodeficiency as the primary diagnosis prior to transplant, and immunosuppression with T-cell antibodies to prevent or treat graft-versus-host disease.[49]

Four main types of PTLD are recognized histologically. Early lesions represent hyperplastic polyclonal proliferations of B cells or plasma cells. Polymorphic PTLD represents polymorphic infiltrates. Monomorphic PTLD is morphologically similar to lymphomas seen in immunocompetent patients and classified similarly to DLBCL, Burkitt lymphoma, plasma cell neoplasms, and T-cell lymphoma. Classic HL-type PTLD is morphologically similar to HL seen in immunocompetent patients.[2]

The risk of developing PTLD is greatest in the first year post-transplant but the median time of onset is only 180 days and 70 to 90 days post–solid organ transplant and stem cell transplant, respectively.[45] The median age of diagnosis is 48 years of age and there is a slight male predominance. Patients often present with fever and malaise and the symptoms may be mistaken for infection.

Although the incidence of pulmonary involvement with PTLD varies depending of the type of allograft, intrathoracic involvement is seen in 69% to 100% of lung, 80% of heart-lung, 32% of heart, 10% to 24% of liver, and 15% of kidney recipients.[50] Lymphadenopathy is seen in up to 60% of patients, but extranodal involvement occurs in more than two-thirds of patients with PTLD due to lung transplant.[2,51] The parenchymal findings of PTLD are similar to those seen with primary pulmonary DLBCL because patients often manifest with multiple pulmonary nodules or masses, usually in a perilymphatic distribution, although isolated lesions can occur. These lesions can greatly vary in both size and morphology (Fig. 15). Although most nodules demonstrate homogenous soft tissue attenuation, surrounding ground-glass halos, internal air bronchograms, and areas of necrosis can occur (Figs. 15 and 16). Patients may also present with solitary or multifocal consolidation with or without associated ground-glass opacity.[50] Septal thickening and pleural effusions can also be seen.[2,52]

There is no established treatment regimen for PTLD but treatment is focused around restoring the recipient's immunity, treating the EBV infection, and removal of neoplastic B cells. Overall, the prognosis of PTLD is variable due

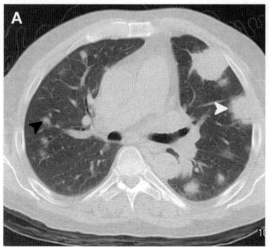
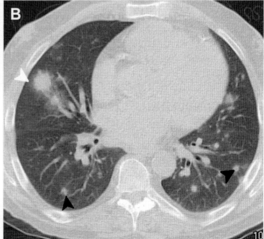

Fig. 15. PTLD in a 55-year-old man 10 months after renal transplant. Axial images (*A*) below the carina and (*B*) at the level of the left atrium shows numerous peribronchovascular and peripheral nodules and masses, many of which demonstrate ground-glass halos (*white arrowheads*). Air bronchograms are seen in many of the nodules and masses but are most conspicuous through the smaller nodules (*black arrowheads*). Wedge resection of a cluster of nodules and masses in the left upper lobe demonstrated polymorphic proliferation of B cells. The patient responded well to therapy and is still alive 9 years after this scan.

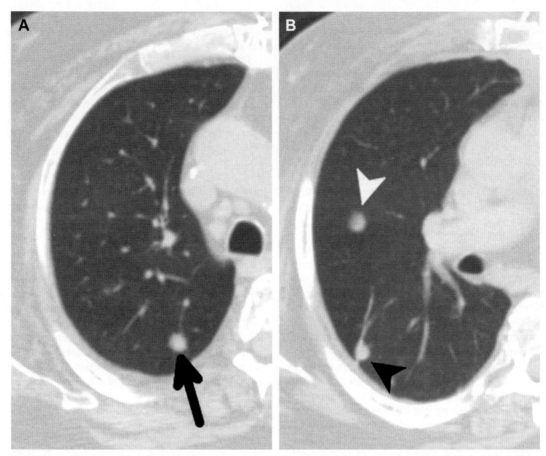

Fig. 16. PTLD in a 52-year-old man 11 months after heart-lung transplantation. Axial CT image (*A*) at the level of the aortic arch and (*B*) through the midlung zone shows scattered small nodules of various morphologies. The nodule in the right lower lobe has a smooth margin (*black arrowhead*); the right upper lobe has a hazy, ill-defined border (*black arrow*); and the nodule adjacent to the minor fissure has a ground-glass halo (*white arrowhead*). Excisional biopsy demonstrated diffuse large B-PTLD.

its variable histology, but median survival rates are approximately 50% to 60% and 30% to 40% at 1 year and 5 years, respectively.[48]

PRIMARY MEDIASTINAL EXTRANODAL LYMPHOMA

In addition to the parenchyma, extranodal lymphoma can occur in the mediastinum. In a majority of instances, these are primary mediastinal large B-cell lymphomas (PMBCLs), which arise from thymic medullary B cells and present as a large anterior mediastinal mass.[53] It accounts for approximately 2% of patients with NHL and tends to involve younger adults (third to fourth decades) than other forms NHL and is more common in women.[54]

Patients often present with a large anterior mediastinal mass that is greater than 10 cm in diameter in approximately two-thirds to

three-quarters of patients (**Fig. 17**).[55] Signs of superior vena cava obstruction are seen in up to 50%, which surprisingly, is a rare finding in patients with HL.[56] Local invasion is common and can be seen in the lung, pericardium, chest wall, and pleura.[54,57,58] Pleural and pericardial effusions are each present in approximately one-third of patients.[59] Despite its local aggressive nature, distant spread is uncommon at time of presentation.

PMBCL shares several histologic and clinical features with nodular sclerosing HL, including similar genetic mutations, prominent fibrosis, younger age of presentation, and the findings of an anterior mediastinal mass.[27,54,60] PMBCL, however, lacks Reed-Sternberg cells and tumor markers differ.

Although PMBCL has been historically associated with a poor prognosis, various chemotherapeutic regiments followed by mediastinal radiation therapy have improved 5-year survival

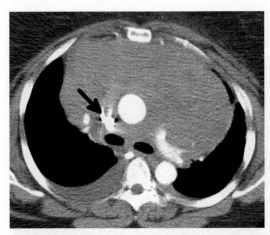

Fig. 17. PMBCL in a 32-year-old woman presenting with facial swelling. Axial CT image shows a large anterior mediastinal mass surrounding the aorta and pulmonary artery. The superior vena cava is narrowed (*arrow*). Although HL was suspected, biopsy showed PMBCL.

to 65%.[21] Newer studies have shown that the addition of rituximab can improve 5-year survival up to 90%.[61–63]

PRIMARY PLEURAL LYMPHOMA

Malignant involvement of the pleura in patients with NHL is not uncommon and can be seen in 6% to 20% of patients (**Fig. 18**).[64–66] Pleural involvement is most commonly seen in patients with DLBCL and is secondary to either lymphatic obstruction by tumor cells or direct extension of tumor into the pleura.[67,68] In rare instances,

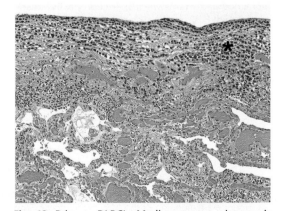

Fig. 18. Primary DLBCL. Medium-power microscopic image (original magnification, ×100; hematoxylin-eosin stain) of lung demonstrates pleural invasion (*asterisk*) by DLBCL due to direct extension of neoplasm.

however, lymphoma may arise from the pleural space. Pleural effusion lymphoma (PEL) is a rare form of HIV-associated DLBCL characterized by lymphomatous fluid in mesothelial lined spaces, such as the pleura, pericardium, and peritoneum (**Fig. 19**).[69,70] A vast majority of patients are HIV positive and many have AIDS and preexisting Kaposi sarcoma. By definition, patients with PEL must be infected with human herpesvirus (HHV)-8.[71]

Another rare form of primary pleural lymphoma was initially termed, pyothorax-associated lymphoma (PAL). The term PAL was coined because first described in patients with chronic pyothorax due to tuberculous pleuritis or artificial pneumothorax for treatment of pulmonary tuberculosis.[72] On average, patients are 64 years of age and present 20 to 64 years after the initial history of pyothorax.[73] PAL is strongly associated with the EBV. PAL was classified as a unique form of lymphoma in the 2004 WHO classification. The development of PAL is not isolated, however, to patients with pyothorax because histologically identical lymphomas have been seen in the pleural space and throughout the body in EBV-positive patients with others causes of chronic inflammation, such as surgical meshes, metallic implants, and osteomyelitis.[74,75] Therefore, in 2008, this form of pleural lymphoma was reclassified by the WHO as DLBCL associated with chronic inflammation.

Because most cases are due to chronic pyothorax, CT often shows invasive pleural soft tissue masses directly adjacent to a coexistent empyema cavity with pleural calcification. Masses can grow circumferentially along the pleural surface or show growth outside the pleural space into the chest wall, diaphragm, mediastinum, lung, pericardium, or bone.[76]

SUMMARY

Primary extranodal lymphomas of the thorax are uncommon diseases that can involve the lung, mediastinum, or pleura. Although the appearance can vary, PPL should be considered in the presence of nonresolving peribronchovascular nodules, masses, or consolidation, often with air bronchograms. Although a similar finding in a post-transplant patient can often mimic infection, PTLD should also be considered in this subset of patients. Primary mediastinal B-cell lymphoma can mimic HL by presenting as an isolated large anterior mediastinal mass in a young adult but often leads to SVC obstruction, a rare finding in patients with HL. Primary pleural lymphomas are

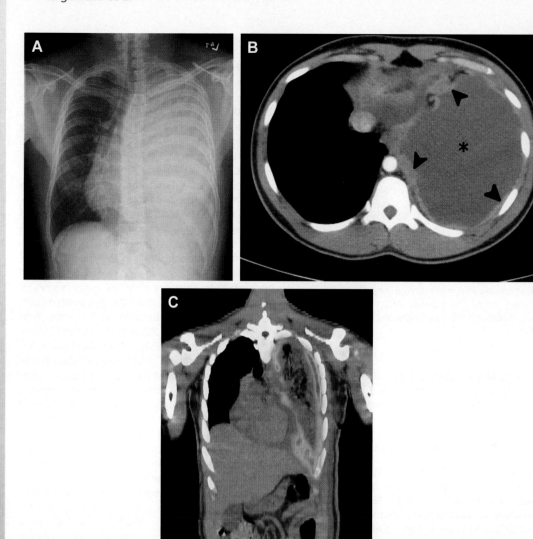

Fig. 19. PEL in a 32-year-old HIV-positive and HHV-8 positive man from Liberia who presented to the emergency department with shortness of breath. (*A*) Posteroanterior radiograph shows a very large left pleural effusion creating mediastinal shift to the right. (*B*) Axial CT image through the lung bases shows the very large left pleural effusion (*asterisk*). There is associated circumferential left pleural nodularity (*arrowheads*). (*C*) Coronal PET image obtained after chest tube placement shows circumferential left pleural FDG uptake. The remainder of the examination was normal.

exceedingly rare and, similar to PTLD, are associated with concomitant viral infections. Although imaging plays an important role in the diagnosis and follow-up of these patients, pathologic diagnosis is vital because the imaging manifestations often are nonspecific in addition to the fact that monoclonal and polyclonal proliferations can look identical on imaging but have different treatments and outcomes.

REFERENCES

1. American Cancer Society. Cancer facts and figures 2015. Atlanta (GA): American Cancer Society; 2015.

2. Hare SS, Souza CA, Bain G, et al. The radiological spectrum of pulmonary lymphoproliferative disease. Br J Radiol 2012;85(1015):848–64.

3. Cadranel J, Wislez M, Antoine M. Primary pulmonary lymphoma. Eur Respir J 2002;20(3):750–62.

4. Poletti V, Ravaglia C, Tomassetti S, et al. Lymphoproliferative lung disorders: clinicopathological aspects. Eur Respir Rev 2013;22(130): 427–36.

5. Ferraro P, Trastek VF, Adlakha H, et al. Primary non-Hodgkin's lymphoma of the lung. Ann Thorac Surg 2000;69(4):993–7.

6. Kim JH, Lee SH, Park J, et al. Primary pulmonary non-Hodgkin's lymphoma. Jpn J Clin Oncol 2004; 34(9):510–4.

7. Herbert A, Walters MT, Cawley MI, et al. Lympho-cytic interstitial pneumonia identified as lymphoma of mucosa associated lymphoid tissue. J Pathol 1985;146(2):129–38.

8. Cohen SM, Petryk M, Varma M, et al. Non-Hodgkin's lymphoma of mucosa-associated lymphoid tissue. Oncologist 2006;11(10):1100–17.

9. Travis WD, Galvin JR. Non-neoplastic pulmonary lymphoid lesions. Thorax 2001;56(12):964–71.

10. Nicholson AG, Wotherspoon AC, Diss TC, et al. Reactive pulmonary lymphoid disorders. Histopa-thology 1995;26(5):405–12.

11. Parissis H. Forty years literature review of primary lung lymphoma. J Cardiothorac Surg 2011;6:23.

12. Zinzani PL, Martelli M, Poletti V, et al. Practice guidelines for the management of extranodal non-Hodgkin's lym-phomas of adult non-immunodeficient patients. Part I: primary lung and mediastinal lymphomas. A project of the Italian Society of Hematology, the Italian Society of Experimental Hematology and the Italian Group for Bone Marrow Transplantation. Haematologica 2008; 93(9):1364–71.

13. Lluch-Garcia R, Briones-Gomez A, Castellano EM, et al. Primary pulmonary Hodgkin's lymphoma. Can Respir J 2010;17(6):e106–8.

14. Katzenstein AL, Doxtader E, Narendra S. Lympho-matoid granulomatosis: insights gained over 4 de-cades. Am J Surg Pathol 2010;34(12):e35–48.

15. Sammassimo S, Pruneri G, Andreola G, et al. A retrospective international study on primary extra-nodal marginal zone lymphoma of the lung (BALT lymphoma) on behalf of International Extranodal Lymphoma Study Group (IELSG). Hematol Oncol 2015. [Epub ahead of print].

16. Bende RJ, van Maldegem F, van Noesel CJ. Chronic inflammatory disease, lymphoid tissue neogenesis and extranodal marginal zone B-cell lymphomas. Haematologica 2009;94(8):1109–23.

17. Routsias JG, Goules JD, Charalampakis G, et al. Malignant lymphoma in primary Sjogren's syndrome: an update on the pathogenesis and treatment. Semin Arthritis Rheum 2013;43(2):178–86.

18. Smedby KE, Baecklund E, Askling J. Malignant lym-phomas in autoimmunity and inflammation: a review of risks, risk factors, and lymphoma characteristics. Cancer Epidemiol Biomarkers Prev 2006;15(11): 2069–77.

19. Kurtin PJ, Myers JL, Adlakha H, et al. Pathologic and clinical features of primary pulmonary extranodal marginal zone B-cell lymphoma of MALT type. Am J Surg Pathol 2001;25(8):997–1008.

20. Bernatsky S, Ramsey-Goldman R, Rajan R, et al. Non-Hodgkin's lymphoma in systemic lupus erythematosus. Ann Rheum Dis 2005;64(10): 1507–9.

21. Mariette X, Cazals-Hatem D, Warszawki J, et al. Lymphomas in rheumatoid arthritis patients treated with methotrexate: a 3-year prospective study in France. Blood 2002;99(11):3909–15.

22. Suarez F, Lortholary O, Hermine O, et al. Infection-associated lymphomas derived from marginal zone B cells: a model of antigen-driven lymphoprolifera-tion. Blood 2006;107(8):3034–44.

23. Bae YA, Lee KS, Han J, et al. Marginal zone B-cell lymphoma of bronchus-associated lymphoid tissue: imaging findings in 21 patients. Chest 2008;133(2): 433–40.

24. Zhang WD, Guan YB, Li CX, et al. Pulmonary mucosa-associated lymphoid tissue lymphoma: com-puted tomography and (1)(8)F fluorodeoxyglucose-positron emission tomography/computed tomography imaging findings and follow-up. J Comput Assist Tomogr 2011;35(5):608–13.

25. Kinsely BL, Mastey LA, Mergo PJ, et al. Pulmonary mucosa-associated lymphoid tissue lymphoma: CT and pathologic findings. AJR Am J Roentgenol 1999;172(5):1321–6.

26. King LJ, Padley SP, Wotherspoon AC, et al. Pulmo-nary MALT lymphoma: imaging findings in 24 cases. Eur Radiol 2000;10(12):1932–8.

27. Ferry JA. Extranodal lymphoma. Arch Pathol Lab Med 2008;132(4):565–78.

28. Bacon CM, Du MQ, Dogan A. Mucosa-associated lymphoid tissue (MALT) lymphoma: a practical guide for pathologists. J Clin Pathol 2007;60(4): 361–72.

29. Lim JK, Lacy MQ, Kurtin PJ, et al. Pulmonary mar-ginal zone lymphoma of MALT type as a cause of lo-calised pulmonary amyloidosis. J Clin Pathol 2001; 54(8):642–6.

30. Desai SR, Nicholson AG, Stewart S, et al. Benign pulmonary lymphocytic infiltration and amyloidosis: computed tomographic and patho-logic features in three cases. J Thorac Imaging 1997;12(3):215–20.

31. Satani T, Yokose T, Kaburagi T, et al. Amyloid depo-sition in primary pulmonary marginal zone B-cell lymphoma of mucosa-associated lymphoid tissue. Pathol Int 2007;57(11):746–50.

32. Deutsch AJ, Aigelsreiter A, Staber PB, et al. MALT lymphoma and extranodal diffuse large B-cell lymphoma are targeted by aberrant somatic hypermutation. Blood 2007;109(8): 3500–4.

33. Cadranel J, Naccache J, Wislez M, et al. Pulmonary malignancies in the immunocompromised patient. Respiration 1999;66(4):289–309.

34. Neri N, Jesus Nambo M, Aviles A. Diffuse large B-cell lymphoma primary of lung. Hematology 2011;16(2):110–2.

35. Dunleavy K, Roschewski M, Wilson WH. Lymphoma-toid granulomatosis and other Epstein-Barr virus associated lymphoproliferative processes. Curr Hematol Malig Rep 2012;7(3):208–15.

36. Liebow AA, Carrington CR, Friedman PJ. Lymphomatoid granulomatosis. Hum Pathol 1972;3:457–558.

37. Katzenstein AL, Peiper SC. Detection of Epstein-Barr virus genomes in lymphomatoid granulomatosis: analysis of 29 cases by the polymerase chain reaction technique. Mod Pathol 1990;3(4): 435–41.

38. Colby TV. Current histological diagnosis of lymphomatoid granulomatosis. Mod Pathol 2012; 25(Suppl 1):S39–42.

39. Roschewski M, Wilson WH. Lymphomatoid granulomatosis. Cancer J 2012;18(5):469–74.

40. Vahid B, Salerno DA, Marik PE. Lymphomatoid granulomatosis: a rare cause of multiple pulmonary nodules. Respir Care 2008;53(9):1227–9.

41. Katzenstein AL, Carrington CB, Liebow AA. Lymphomatoid granulomatosis: a clinicopathologic study of 152 cases. Cancer 1979;43(1):360–73.

42. Lee JS, Tuder R, Lynch DA. Lymphomatoid granulomatosis: radiologic features and pathologic correlations. AJR Am J Roentgenol 2000;175(5): 1335–9.

43. Frazier AA, Rosado-de-Christenson ML, Galvin JR, et al. Pulmonary angiitis and granulomatosis: radiologic-pathologic correlation. Radiographics 1998;18(3):687–710 [quiz: 727].

44. Paya CV, Fung JJ, Nalesnik MA, et al. Epstein-Barr virus-induced posttransplant lymphoproliferative disorders. ASTS/ASTP EBV-PTLD Task Force and The Mayo Clinic Organized International Consensus Development Meeting. Transplantation 1999;68(10): 1517–25.

45. Loren AW, Porter DL, Stadtmauer EA, et al. Posttransplant lymphoproliferative disorder: a review. Bone Marrow Transplant 2003;31(3):145–55.

46. Mucha K, Foroncewicz B, Ziarkiewicz-Wroblewska B, et al. Post-transplant lymphoproliferative disorder in view of the new WHO classification: a more rational approach to a protean disease? Nephrol Dial Transplant 2010;25(7):2089–98.

47. Issa NC, Fishman JA. Infectious complications of antilymphocyte therapies in solid organ transplantation. Clin Infect Dis 2009;48(6):772–86.

48. Jacobson CA, LaCasce AS. Lymphoma: risk and response after solid organ transplant. Oncology (Williston Park) 2010;24(10):936–44.

49. Gottschalk S, Rooney CM, Heslop HE. Post-transplant lymphoproliferative disorders. Annu Rev Med 2005;56:29–44.

50. Borhani AA, Hosseinzadeh K, Almusa O, et al. Imaging of posttransplantation lymphoproliferative disorder after solid organ transplantation. Radiographics 2009; 29(4):981–1000 [discussion: 1000–2].

51. LaCasce AS. Post-transplant lymphoproliferative disorders. Oncologist 2006;11(6):674–80.

52. Collins J, Muller NL, Leung AN, et al. Epstein-Barr-virus-associated lymphoproliferative disease of the lung: CT and histologic findings. Radiology 1998;208(3):749–59.

53. Martelli M, Di Rocco A, Russo E, et al. Primary mediastinal lymphoma: diagnosis and treatment options. Expert Rev Hematol 2015;8(2):173–86.

54. Savage KJ. Rare B-cell lymphomas: primary mediastinal, intravascular, and primary effusion lymphoma. Cancer Treat Res 2008;142:243–64.

55. Martelli M, Ferreri AJ, Johnson P. Primary mediastinal large B-cell lymphoma. Crit Rev Oncol Hematol 2008;68(3):256–63.

56. Wilson LD, Detterbeck FC, Yahalom J. Clinical practice. Superior vena cava syndrome with malignant causes. N Engl J Med 2007;356(18):1862–9.

57. Todeschini G, Secchi S, Morra E, et al. Primary mediastinal large B-cell lymphoma (PMLBCL): long-term results from a retrospective multicentre Italian experience in 138 patients treated with CHOP or MACOP-B/VACOP-B. Br J Cancer 2004; 90(2):372–6.

58. Johnson PW, Davies AJ. Primary mediastinal B-cell lymphoma. Hematology Am Soc Hematol Educ Program 2008;349–58.

59. Shaffer K, Smith D, Kirn D, et al. Primary mediastinal large-B-cell lymphoma: radiologic findings at presentation. AJR Am J Roentgenol 1996;167(2): 425–30.

60. Savage KJ, Monti S, Kutok JL, et al. The molecular signature of mediastinal large B-cell lymphoma differs from that of other diffuse large B-cell lymphomas and shares features with classical Hodgkin lymphoma. Blood 2003;102(12):3871–9.

61. Avigdor A, Sirotkin T, Kedmi M, et al. The impact of R-VACOP-B and interim FDG-PET/CT on outcome in primary mediastinal large B cell lymphoma. Ann Hematol 2014;93(8):1297–304.

62. Ceriani L, Martelli M, Zinzani PL, et al. Utility of baseline 18FDG-PET/CT functional parameters in defining prognosis of primary mediastinal (thymic) large B-cell lymphoma. Blood 2015; 126(8):950–6.

63. Martelli M, Ceriani L, Zucca E, et al. [18F]fluorodeoxyglucose positron emission tomography predicts survival after chemoimmunotherapy for primary mediastinal large B-cell lymphoma: results of the International Extranodal Lymphoma Study Group IELSG-26 Study. J Clin Oncol 2014;32(17):1769–75.

64. Johnston WW. The malignant pleural effusion. A review of cytopathologic diagnoses of 584 specimens from 472 consecutive patients. Cancer 1985;56(4): 905–9.

65. Manoharan A, Pitney WR, Schonell ME, et al. Intrathoracic manifestations in non-Hodgkin's lymphoma. Thorax 1979;34(1):29–32.

66. Elis A, Blickstein D, Mulchanov I, et al. Pleural effusion in patients with non-Hodgkin's lymphoma: a case-controlled study. Cancer 1998;83(8):1607–11.

67. Vega F, Padula A, Valbuena JR, et al. Lymphomas involving the pleura: a clinicopathologic study of 34 cases diagnosed by pleural biopsy. Arch Pathol Lab Med 2006;130(10):1497–502.

68. Berkman N, Breuer R. Pulmonary involvement in lymphoma. Respir Med 1993;87(2):85–92.

69. Chen YB, Rahemtullah A, Hochberg E. Primary effusion lymphoma. Oncologist 2007;12(5):569–76.

70. Wakely PE Jr, Menezes G, Nuovo GJ. Primary effusion lymphoma: cytopathologic diagnosis using in situ molecular genetic analysis for human herpesvirus 8. Mod Pathol 2002;15(9):944–50.

71. Nador RG, Cesarman E, Chadburn A, et al. Primary effusion lymphoma: a distinct clinicopathologic entity associated with the Kaposi's sarcoma-associated herpes virus. Blood 1996;88(2):645–56.

72. Aozasa K. Pyothorax-associated lymphoma. J Clin Exp Hematop 2006;46(1):5–10.

73. Nakatsuka S, Yao M, Hoshida Y, et al. Pyothorax-associated lymphoma: a review of 106 cases. J Clin Oncol 2002;20(20):4255–60.

74. Fujimoto M, Haga H, Okamoto M, et al. EBV-associated diffuse large B-cell lymphoma arising in the chest wall with surgical mesh implant. Pathol Int 2008;58(10):668–71.

75. Sanchez-Gonzalez B, Garcia M, Montserrat F, et al. Diffuse large B-cell lymphoma associated with chronic inflammation in metallic implant. J Clin Oncol 2013;31(10):e148–51.

76. Ueda T, Andreas C, Itami J, et al. Pyothorax-associated lymphoma: imaging findings. AJR Am J Roentgenol 2010;194(1):76–84.

Cardiac Lymphoma

Jean Jeudy, MD[a], Allen P. Burke, MD[b], Aletta Ann Frazier, MD[a,c],*

KEYWORDS

- Primary cardiac lymphoma • Diffuse large B-cell lymphoma • Primary effusion lymphoma
- Posttransplant lymphoproliferative disorder (PTLD) • Cardiac neoplasia

KEY POINTS

- Primary cardiac lymphoma is rare, but secondary cardiac lymphoma occurs in almost 25% of patients with disseminated lymphoma.
- Cardiac lymphoma usually affects older immunocompetent individuals, but a subset occurs in immunocompromised patients, including allograft recipients and human immunodeficiency virus-AIDS patients.
- Lymphoma often involves the right side of the heart, especially the right atrium. Epicardial and pericardial infiltration with pericardial effusion is typical.
- Clinical complications reflect the underlying anatomic site impacted by tumor and include conduction abnormalities, pericardial effusion ($\pm$ tamponade), congestive heart failure, angina, and superior vena caval syndrome.
- Treatment includes chemotherapy, variably combined with radiotherapy, but prognosis remains poor. Surgery is performed for palliation in select cases.

INTRODUCTION

Secondary cardiac involvement by lymphoma is discovered in almost 25% of patients with disseminated disease.[1,2] Primary cardiac lymphoma (PCL), on the other hand, is rare and accounts for less than 2% of all resected primary cardiac tumors and 0.5% of extranodal lymphomas at autopsy.[1,3–5] The incidence of PCL is thought to be increasing in recent years because of the evolution of sophisticated imaging modalities, diagnostic testing, and surgical techniques.[1,3,6] In addition, there is more frequent recognition of cardiac lymphoma in immunocompromised patients.[1,6]

Cardiac lymphomas are infiltrative, intramural, and epicardial lesions that may be singular or multiple, and the pericardium is involved in about a third of cases.[3] The imaging features of primary and secondary cardiac lymphoma are largely shared, although many studies suggest that PCL favors the right side of the heart.[6] PCL tends to involve the right-sided cardiac chambers, especially the right atrium, and is often multifocal.[1] The superior vena cava (SVC) is involved in up to 25% of cases.[6] Extracardiac sites of lymphoma are actively sought during diagnostic evaluation, including the mediastinum and bone marrow, in order to clarify whether the cardiac lymphoma is primary or secondary.[1,7]

It must be acknowledged that the diagnosis of PCL has various shades of meaning. The diagnostic criteria have gradually broadened since its earliest description in the 1930s.[6] If lymphoma exclusively involves the heart or pericardium, then the diagnosis is straightforward. In some cases, however, the diagnosis of PCL is assigned if the primary burden of tumor resides

[a] Department of Diagnostic Radiology and Nuclear Medicine, University of Maryland School of Medicine, 22 South Greene Street, Baltimore, MD 21201, USA; [b] Department of Pathology, University of Maryland School of Medicine, Baltimore, MD, USA; [c] American Institute for Radiologic Pathology, 1010 Wayne Avenue, Silver Spring, MD, USA
* Corresponding author. 3942 Washington Street, Kensington, MD 20895.
E-mail address: afrazier@acr.org

Radiol Clin N Am 54 (2016) 689–710
http://dx.doi.org/10.1016/j.rcl.2016.03.006
0033-8389/16/$ – see front matter © 2016 Elsevier Inc. All rights reserved.

in the heart or pericardium even if limited extracardiac lymphoma is identified. When the clinical presentation directly reflects the impact of lymphoma on cardiac anatomy or function (including a significant pericardial effusion), this further supports a diagnosis of primary rather than secondary cardiac lymphoma (Box 1).[1,3,6]

Almost all cardiac lymphomas are of B-cell lineage and most often (80%) diffuse large B-cell lymphoma (DLBCL), a subtype of non-Hodgkin lymphoma.[3,4] PCL usually occurs in immunocompetent adults (mean age 60 years; range 12–86 years) with a male predominance (2:1).[1,6] A subset of cardiac lymphoma is identified in Epstein-Barr virus (EBV)-related lymphoproliferative disorders found in allograft recipients and AIDS patients.[5,8] Cardiac lymphoma and other extranodal lymphomas found in immunocompromised patients are usually high-grade B-cell lymphomas.[1,9] Patients with cardiac or lung transplantation are more likely affected by posttransplant lymphoproliferative disorder (PTLD) (6%) than renal transplant recipients (<1%). Cardiac lymphoma remains very unusual in the setting of PTLD compared with the more common central nervous system (CNS), bone marrow, gastrointestinal tract, and mucocutaneous sites.[1,10]

Primary effusion lymphoma (PEL), formerly termed body cavity lymphoma, is a distinct subtype of lymphoma that may manifest as a malignant pericardial effusion. PEL may arise in the pericardium, peritoneum, or pleural space and represents a liquid phase of lymphoma without extracavitary solid nodal disease.[11] PEL accounts for about 4% of all human immunodeficiency virus (HIV)–associated non-Hodgkin lymphomas and is associated with human herpes virus (HHV)-8 infection and a concomitant diagnosis of Kaposi sarcoma in immunocompromised patients.[1,11,12] PEL is also described in HIV-negative patients who have had solid organ transplantation and are receiving immunosuppressive therapy. In order to help distinguish PEL from a lymphomatous effusion secondary to other forms of non-Hodgkin lymphoma, confirmation of viral infection by HHV-8 in the neoplastic cells is required.[1,11]

An unusual form of cardiac lymphoma occurs in the setting of implanted cardiac devices (including prosthetic valves and synthetic grafts) and is termed fibrin-associated large B-cell lymphoma. The cause is uncertain but may be related to a chronic foreign body inflammatory reaction.[1,3]

CLINICAL PRESENTATION

Dyspnea is the most commonly reported clinical symptom at presentation (64%), followed by constitutional complaints (26%) and chest pain (24%).[6,13,14] Congestive heart failure affects almost half of all patients.[6] Cardiac lymphoma has even been considered an oncologic emergency in scenarios of rapid tumor evolution and advanced organ infiltration. If there is direct infiltration of a coronary artery or ostium, the patient may experience angina.[1]

Cardiac arrhythmias are commonly identified on electrocardiographic (ECG) tracing (affecting 56% of patients according to one study), typically an atrial arrhythmia or atrioventricular block ranging from first to third degree.[6,15] More unusual cases show left or right bundle branch block or ventricular arrhythmia.[6] Sudden death due to cardiac arrhythmia may even be the initial presentation of cardiac lymphoma.[6,16,17]

Certain clinical features of cardiac lymphoma directly reflect the anatomic location of the neoplasm. For example, if there is a significant intramural or intracavitary component of lymphoma within the right atrium or SVC, patients may present with SVC syndrome because of limited venous inflow (5%–8%) (Fig. 1).[6] Right-sided cardiac lesions may be complicated by pulmonary thromboembolism, and left-sided lesions may produce systemic embolism.[18,19] Significant pericardial involvement in cardiac lymphoma is common because of its predilection for the epicardium and is often associated with a pericardial effusion (58%), a pericardial mass (30%), or both (21%) (Fig. 2). Cardiac tamponade is a well-recognized complication in up to 34% of patients with pericardial effusion in cardiac lymphoma; hemopericardium is also reported.[2,6]

Box 1
Diagnostic criteria for cardiac lymphoma

Tissue sampling via direct biopsy, open resection, or pericardial cytology

Malignant lymphoid cells are centered in myocardium and/or pericardium

Clinical presentation reflects tumor's impact on heart and/or pericardium

Extracardiac lymphoma is minimal to nonexistent in primary cardiac lymphoma

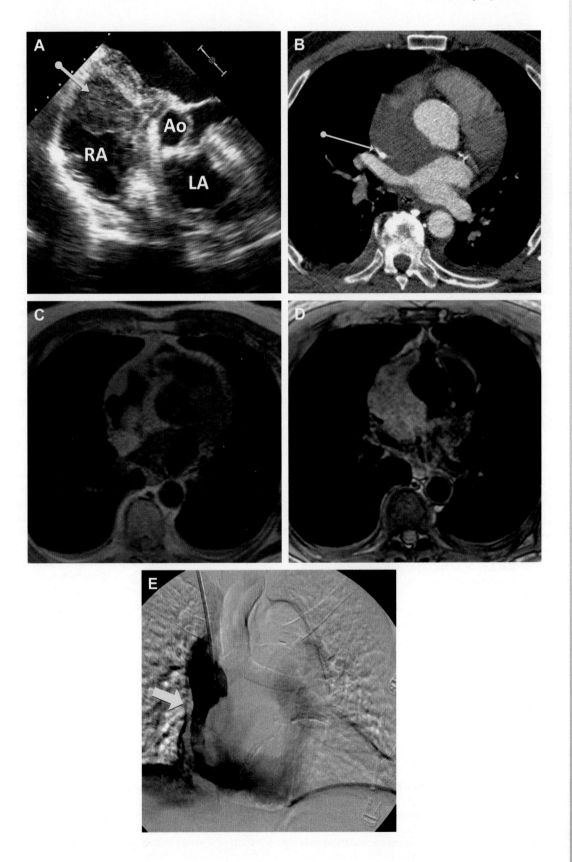

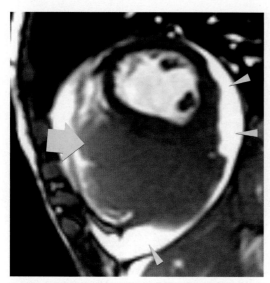

Fig. 2. A 49-year-old woman with cardiac lymphoma. Short axial MR SSFP image demonstrates a large ill-defined mass mildly hyperintense compared with myocardium (*thick arrow*). The mass infiltrates through the myocardium inferiorly into the pericardium and is associated with a large pericardial effusion (*arrowheads*).

DIAGNOSTIC IMAGING

Chest radiography is limited for the detection of cardiac tumor, occasionally revealing nonspecific signs of pleural effusion or cardiomegaly. Transthoracic echocardiography allows for initial noninvasive assessment of cardiac disease and in many cases is the first-line imaging evaluation. However, complementary assessment with cross-sectional imaging is now essential for further characterization of the tumor and the extent of involvement. Both computed tomography (CT) and magnetic resonance (MR) imaging have significantly improved tissue and contrast resolution, allowing for enhanced evaluation of tissue based on attenuation or signal intensity.

Computed Tomography

CT provides excellent anatomic assessment of cardiac lymphoma involvement, primarily due to its high isotropic spatial and temporal resolution. It benefits from fast acquisition time and is a primary alternative in imaging patients with known contraindications to MR or in patients with inadequate images from other noninvasive methods. In addition to delineating the extent of cardiac disease, CT provides a field of view that encompasses the entire chest and thereby optimizes assessment of extracardiac disease.

Computed tomography imaging protocol

The advent of ECG synchronization techniques allows for decreased motion-related artifacts and more precise delineation of cardiac structures. 64-Multidetector CT and higher detector row scanners provide volumetric acquisitions with isotropic image resolution (**Table 1**). Evaluation of cardiac masses can be satisfactorily achieved with 1- to 3-mm-slice collimation with slice overlap for multiplanar reconstruction. A large field of view is essential for adequate evaluation of extracardiac disease and incidental findings. Image parameters should always be tailored to the patient. Kilovoltage may range from 80 to 140 kVp depending on body mass index.[20–22]

Contrast injection protocols should prioritize adequate opacification of right heart structures, particularly to evaluate myocardial invasion. Approximately 60 to 100 mL of nonionic contrast is administered with either a single- or a dual-syringe power injector system. Precontrast and delayed phase imaging may provide additional tissue characterization. Low-dose protocols mitigate the burden of radiation dose with the additional information these phases provide.

The main drawbacks to CT include radiation exposure and the need to give iodinated contrast media. Because cardiac lymphomas have the tendency for right heart invasion, streak artifacts from contrast injection may limit visualization of the tumor morphology.

Computed tomography imaging findings

On CT, cardiac lymphoma classically presents as a variably or poorly enhancing mass typically arising in the right side of the heart with similar prevalence of right atrial and ventricular involvement.[23,24] Extension along the epicardial surface

---

Fig. 1. A 70-year-old man with new onset facial swelling and chest pain. (*A*) Transesophageal echocardiogram with parasternal view reveals a largely intracavitary mass in the right atrium related to the interatrial septum (*arrow*). (*B*) Contrast-enhanced axial CT better depicts the extent of disease and myocardial infiltration. Mass effect on the SVC results in slitlike compression (*arrow*). (*C, D*) Cardiac MR reveals the mass to be isointense to myocardium on T1W (*C*) and T2W (*D*) sequences. (*E*) Conventional angiography demonstrates the extent of SVC compression (*thick arrow*). Cardiac lymphoma was confirmed by biopsy. Ao, aorta; LA, left atrium; RA, right atrium.

Table 1 Imaging protocols: cardiac computed tomography	
Parameter Type	
General specifications	
Collimation	Best spatial resolution for optimal diagnostic assessment will be with CT detector widths <0.625 mm
Pitch	Adaptive dependent on heart rate
kV	80–140 kV
mA	Modulation techniques should be used and tailored for the patient
Cardiac gating	
ECG-gating	Prospective ECG-triggered or retrospective ECG-gated CT imaging using tube modulation techniques
Reconstruction slice thickness	Thin sections ≤1 mm Thick reconstructions at 2–4 mm
Cardiac phases	If acquired with retrospective technique, 2-mm-thick images every 10% for 10 phases; otherwise, end-diastolic phases with prospective triggering
Contrast administration	
Contrast parameters	Test bolus vs bolus tracking
Contrast type	Nonionic iodinated contrast at least 300 mg/mL
Contrast volume	60–100 mL
Saline flush	30 mL
Injection rate	4–8 mL/s

Adapted from Abbara S, Arbab-Zadeh A, Callister TQ, et al. SCCT guidelines for performance of coronary computed tomographic angiography: a report of the Society of Cardiovascular Computed Tomography Guidelines Committee. J Cardiovasc Comput Tomogr 2009;3(3):190–204.

of the heart is common, as is encasement of the coronary vessels and the aortic root (**Fig. 3**).[1,25] The mass may be lower in attenuation compared with regional skeletal muscle. PCLs are less likely to involve the valves, although isolated cases have been reported.[4,26,27] Both pericardial thickening and effusion may be observed in both primary and secondary forms of cardiac lymphoma involvement and in some cases may be the predominant imaging finding. Pericardial effusions can be large and in severe cases may result in cardiac tamponade (**Fig. 4**).[28–31]

MR Imaging

Despite the greater availability of other imaging modalities, cardiac MR is the preferred imaging modality for cardiac masses because of its superior soft tissue characterization, high temporal resolution, multiplanar imaging capabilities, and unrestricted field of view.[32]

MR imaging protocol
With the variety and complexity of MR sequence options, a coordinated protocol optimizing diagnostic information, scan time, and patient

comfort should be sought (**Table 2**).[33] Most evaluations are sufficiently performed at a field strength of 1.5 T. Conventional imaging in the axial plane with T1 and T2 techniques provides the most fundamental evaluation. Steady-state free precession (SSFP) sequences in the axial plane also provide excellent depiction of the myocardium, blood pool, and adjacent soft tissue. The SSFP technique has high spatial and temporal resolution, contains both T1 and T2 properties, but is skewed more toward T2-weighting.

Beyond morphologic evaluation of the mass, tumor vascularity and perfusion also can be characterized after bolus administration of gadolinium and subsequent assessment of both first-pass perfusion and late gadolinium enhancement (LGE). First-pass imaging is performed with a T1-weighted (T1W) gradient echo technique during the dynamic administration of intravenous contrast, allowing global assessment of vascularity and necrosis. The prescribed slices should focus on the most significant sections of the mass to ensure adequate visualization. Three-dimensional volumetric breath-hold T1

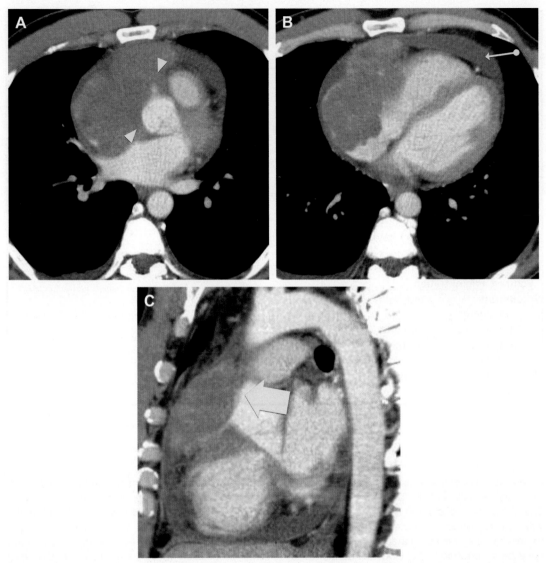

Fig. 3. A 40-year-old man with chest pain and ST elevation on ECG. (*A, B*) Contrast-enhanced axial CT images demonstrate a large, mildly heterogeneous mass infiltrating the wall of the right heart and epicardial surface. Encasement of aortic root and coronary vessels by tumor also observed (*arrowheads*). Moderate pericardial effusion is present (*arrow*). (*C*) Sagittal multiplanar reformat (MPR) further demonstrates obstruction of the right ventricular outflow tract (RVOT) due to encroaching lymphoma (*thick arrow*).

fat-saturated sequences (volumetric interpolated breath-hold examination [VIBE]) may be obtained immediately after perfusion to provide global post-contrast assessment of the chest.[22] Late gadolinium sequences are obtained 10 minutes after contrast administration with an inversion time set to null the myocardium (typically 200–300 milliseconds). An additional delayed sequence may be obtained with an extended inversion time (500–600 milliseconds) to assess for surrounding or associated thrombus.

MR imaging findings
The most distinctive advantage of MR is the ability to characterize tissue with or without administration of intravenous contrast. The different T1 and T2 properties of tissues help to differentiate normal from pathologic tissue. Prior studies suggest that because malignant cells have a higher concentration of free intracellular water content and a greater degree of surrounding interstitial edema, it should follow that malignant lesions would also have longer T1 and T2 relaxation

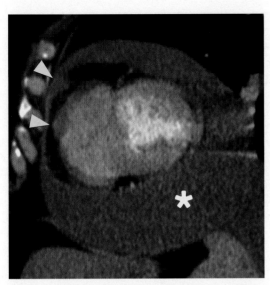

Fig. 4. Cardiac lymphoma with predominant pericardial involvement. Short-axis MPR of a contrast-enhanced chest CT shows a large pericardial effusion (*asterisk*). Cardiac tamponade was revealed on transthoracic echocardiography. There is subtle soft tissue nodularity along the pericardium as well as a small soft tissue mass invading the anterior right heart border (*arrowheads*). Cardiac lymphoma was diagnosed by pericardial fluid cytology.

times when compared with benign abnormality (**Fig. 5**).[20,34,35]

Although cardiac lymphomas may have a variable appearance on MR, they are commonly hypointense on T1W MR sequences and hyperintense on T2-weighted (T2W) sequences.[36,37] The variable signal intensity may be determined by the cellularity of the tumor. For CNS lymphomas, the increase in T2 signal relates to necrosis, although this has not been specifically characterized in cardiac lymphoma.[35,38] Cardiac lymphomas are less likely to have components of hemorrhage or necrosis than sarcomas (**Fig. 6**).

SSFP sequences are the most relied on technique for cardiac MR imaging and provide excellent contrast differentiation between the myocardium and blood pool without contrast. Cine imaging using SSFP technique further depicts dynamic processes, thus allowing for better assessment of tumor mobility and tumor point of attachment as well as its relationship with adjacent cardiac structures.[24,39,40]

Intravenous contrast administration adds additional characterization, although patterns may vary from homogeneous to heterogeneous enhancement (**Fig. 7**). Pericardial effusion can be

seen readily on prior T2W and SSFP sequences. The addition of intravenous contrast may delineate pericardial nodularity, inflammation, and enhancement. Extracardiac lymphadenopathy in the mediastinum may be identified in the setting of systemic disease.

LGE imaging with nulling of normal myocardium has evolved primarily for depicting ischemic disease but also may identify the extent of cardiac masses. There are no characteristic appearances of cardiac lymphoma on LGE sequences. Given that gadolinium is an extracellular agent, the presence of LGE most often correlates to tumor cellularity in the initial - evaluation and areas of myocardial fibrosis in the after-therapeutic setting (**Fig. 8**).[20,32]

Cardiac lymphomas often have adjacent thrombus, which may be difficult to differentiate on other sequences. Performing LGE sequences with an extended inversion time facilitates differentiation between tumor and thrombus. Normal myocardium and even tumor have varying amounts of vascularity, whereas thrombus is characteristically avascular. On first-pass images, lack of contrast enhancement within a thrombus readily distinguishes it from normal or neoplastic tissue. At inversion times optimized for nulling of the myocardium during assessment for LGE (200–350 milliseconds), thrombus may be indistinguishable from adjacent myocardium or tumor. However, at extended inversion times (500–600 milliseconds), the signal from both myocardium and tumor will increase because of residual gadolinium in their extracellular space. Adjacent or adherent thrombus, which is avascular and without the presence of gadolinium in its extracellular space, will remain dark in signal at these extended inversion times. Weinsaft and colleagues[41] investigated the accuracy of this technique and found that LGE detected intracardiac thrombus in 7% (n = 55) of patients compared with cine cardiac MR imaging in 4.7% (37 patients; $P<.005$) (**Fig. 9**).

NUCLEAR MEDICINE IMAGING

The utility of nuclear medicine techniques for the noninvasive assessment of cardiac lymphomas has largely been limited to assessment of treatment response, although more robust diagnostic applications are being investigated. Gallium-67 uptake has been demonstrated in the heart and pericardium as well as in lymphoma. These findings are nonspecific, although marked accumulation within the heart without evidence of

Table 2
Imaging protocols: cardiac MR imaging

Sequence (Sequences Should Match in Anatomic Coverage to Ensure Optimal Multi-sequence Comparison)	
Precontrast	
T1W fast spin echo without/with fat suppression	Axial acquisition with attention to extent of myocardial invasion and extracardiac involvement
T2W, short tau inversion recovery with fat suppression	Axial acquisition to assess myocardial edema
SSFP	Best sequence for detection of mass infiltration into the myocardium and regional tissues; cine images allow for dynamic assessment of tumor properties • Axial non cine • Cine SSFP in short, horizontal long, and vertical long axis
Contrast administration	
Gadolinium chelate (0.1–0.2 mmol/kg)	Injection rate 3–7 mL/s
Postcontrast	
First-pass perfusion (gradient echo/echo planar)	• At least one slice through the mass to assess vascularity
Postcontrast T1 (fast spin echo vs VIBE)	• Match anatomic coverage with precontrast sequences • Assess for areas of tumor enhancement • Assess extracardiac involvement
LGE	Approximately 10 min after gadolinium administration; 2-dimensional segmented inversion recovery GRE or SSFP • Typical evaluation with TI = 250–350 ms • Differentiate thrombus with TI = 600 ms

Adapted from Kramer CM, Barkhausen J, Flamm SD, et al. Society for Cardiovascular Magnetic Resonance Board of Trustees Task Force on Standardized Protocols. Standardized cardiovascular magnetic resonance imaging (CMR) protocols, Society for Cardiovascular Magnetic Resonance: Board of Trustees Task Force on standardized protocols. J Cardiovasc Magn Reson 2008;10(1):35.

extracardiac uptake may suggest the diagnosis of cardiac lymphoma.[42,43]

18F-Fluorodeoxyglucose PET with CT (18F-FDG-PET/CT) is reliable in the assessment of lymphoma throughout the body for initial staging and treatment response.[44] The utility of FDG-PET alone for the specific diagnosis of cardiac lymphoma may be challenging due to the physiologic accumulation of radiotracer within the myocardium and the low anatomic resolution of FDG-PET.[45,46] However, in combination with anatomic information from CT, there is improved diagnostic and staging accuracy and improved confidence in interpretation (**Fig. 10**). Involved portions of the heart, pericardium, and pleura may demonstrate intense metabolic activity compared with physiologic uptake. Case reports confirm that cardiac lymphoma is an FDG-avid lesion relative to surrounding myocardium and further suggest that FDG-PET/CT may be a useful imaging modality to monitor treatment response in this disease.[47–51]

RADIOLOGIC DIFFERENTIAL DIAGNOSIS

The main diagnostic considerations for an intramural cardiac mass, particularly one affecting the right heart, are metastatic disease (most commonly from a lung primary), secondary or primary lymphoma, benign primary cardiac neoplasms (eg, atypical atrial myxoma), and a primary cardiac sarcoma such as angiosarcoma (**Box 2, Table 3**). Histologic examination and immunophenotypic studies ultimately distinguish among these neoplasms (**Fig. 11**), but imaging features may also guide the differential diagnosis.[1,52]

Metastatic lung carcinoma, which may involve the heart and pericardium by direct extension or lymphatic or hematogenous dissemination, is

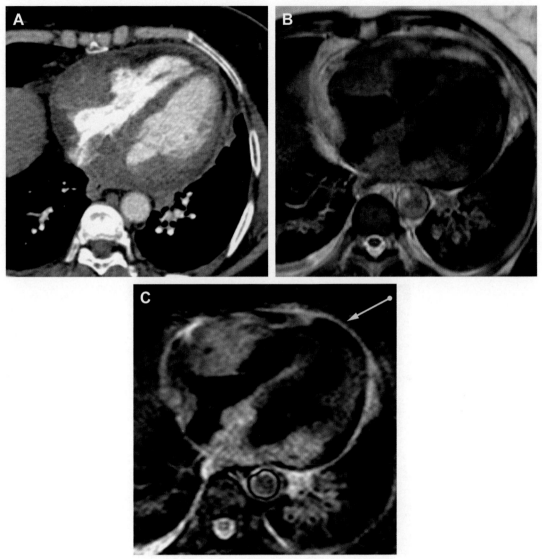

Fig. 5. A 62-year-old patient with dyspnea on exertion and chest pain. (*A*) Contrast-enhanced axial chest CT demonstrates a soft tissue mass broadly infiltrating the right heart. The mass extends along the epicardial surface of the heart to also involve the interatrial septum and left atrium. (*B, C*) Cardiac MR demonstrates the mass to be isointense on T1W (*B*) and slightly hyperintense on T2W (*C*) sequences. Note the prominence in signal delineating pericardial involvement on T2W image (*arrow*).

suggested radiologically when a primary tumor mass is identified in the lung parenchyma.[53,54] Malignant melanoma metastatic to the heart has a prevalence of 46% to 71% in autopsy series and may involve all 4 chambers.[55,56] Whereas cardiac lymphomas are typically hypointense on T1W MR sequences and hyperintense on T2W sequences, melanoma lesions in the heart demonstrate increased signal intensity on both T1- and T2W images compatible with blood and melanin content.[57]

Cardiac sarcomas comprise a diverse group of mesenchymal tumors that may be difficult to discern from cardiac lymphomas (**Fig. 12**).[1,56] Angiosarcoma, the most common differentiated form of cardiac sarcoma, shares with lymphoma the propensity for the right atrium and pericardial involvement with effusion. However, a cardiac sarcoma tends to be more aggressive than cardiac lymphoma. For example, angiosarcoma may demonstrate central necrosis, involve extensive areas of the heart, and penetrate cardiac valves

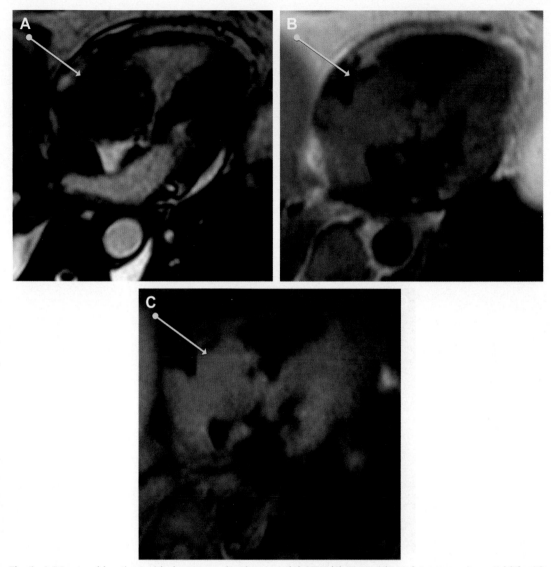

Fig. 6. A 54-year-old patient with dyspnea and orthopnea. (*A*) SSFP. (*B*) T1W without fat suppression, and (*C*) with fat suppression depicting infiltration of the right heart by cardiac lymphoma (*arrows*). The images demonstrate both intramural and intracavitary components. The mass is isointense to the myocardium on T1W image (*B*) without evidence of necrosis.

and the great vessels.[4,23,36,58–61] Although angiosarcoma typically displays prominent contrast enhancement on both CT and MR imaging, cardiac lymphoma does not display striking enhancement patterns. On contrast-enhanced CT, angiosarcoma appears as a heterogeneous nodular mass containing areas of low attenuation (necrosis) as well as pools of high attenuation (hemorrhage).[62,63] On MR imaging, angiosarcoma appears largely isointense on T1W sequences with smaller areas of high T1 signal (reflecting blood

products) and areas of absent signal (representing flow voids within dilated vascular channels). Angiosarcoma demonstrates high signal on T2W sequences and intense postgadolinium enhancement along vascular channels described as a "sunray pattern."[64,65] These CT and MR imaging characteristics overall are not typical of cardiac lymphoma and help to distinguish between these 2 neoplasms.

The presence of a pericardial effusion in the setting of a cardiac mass, particularly with

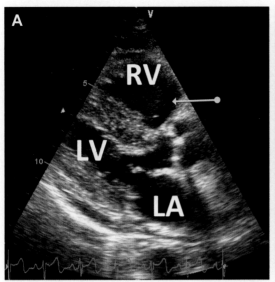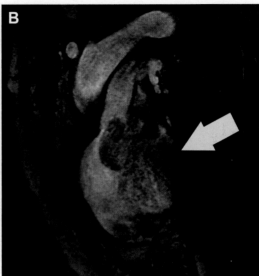

Fig. 7. An 80-year-old woman with dyspnea, chest pain, and bilateral lower extremity edema. (*A*) Echocardiography demonstrates vague echogenicity in the RVOT resulting in a pressure gradient across the pulmonary valve (*thin arrow*). (*B*) T1W postcontrast cardiac MR in oblique sagittal view confirms a mildly heterogeneously enhancing tumor that infiltrates the right ventricle and extends into the RVOT (*thick arrow*). LA, left atrium; LV, left ventricle; RV, right ventricle.

demonstrated pericardial enhancement or nodularity, suggests an associated malignant pericardial process. Nevertheless, there is a broad differential diagnosis for pericardial effusion even in the setting of cardiac malignancy. Pericardial malignancy relies on pericardial fluid cytology for definitive diagnosis and is usually the consequence of neoplastic invasion via lymphatic channels.[53] Pericardial effusion in the setting of cardiac lymphoma may represent direct neoplastic involvement (most likely via epicardial to pericardial spread) or the consequence of lymphatic obstruction by the tumor.[1,66]

Special Considerations in the Immunocompromised Patient

The imaging manifestations of primary and secondary cardiac lymphomas are identical in immunocompromised and immunocompetent patients. However, given the higher incidence of cardiac involvement with lymphoma in this subset of patients, greater suspicion is warranted. PTLD, a B-cell proliferation induced by EBV infection, may develop in AIDS patients or in patients months to years following solid organ or stem cell transplantation. Although cardiac lymphoma reflects less than 5% of all lymphomas arising in these patients, this still reflects a subgroup of patients at increased risk.[1,67,68] Aside from the typical pericardial effusion that may develop as a result of cardiac lymphomatous involvement, immunocompromised patients may also develop a PEL (**Fig. 13**). As noted above, this diagnosis requires confirmation of neoplastic cell infection by HHV-8.[11,12]

PATHOLOGY

Primary cardiac lymphomas typically occur as multiple masses of firm, white, homogeneous nodules with "fish flesh" consistency on gross inspection. The sites of the heart most often affected by lymphoma are the right atrium, followed by the right ventricle, left ventricle, left atrium, atrial septum, and ventricular septum.[1,8,25,69] Extension of tumor onto valves is unusual, but extension onto the pericardial surfaces frequently occurs. More than one cardiac chamber is involved in more than 75% of cases.

Cardiac lymphomas are usually B-cell neoplasms, most frequently DLBCL, followed by follicular lymphoma and Burkitt lymphoma (**Fig. 14**). In a series of 40 PCLs in immunocompetent patients, 37 were of B-cell lineage, 2 cases were of T-cell lineage, and one was not determined.[70] A more

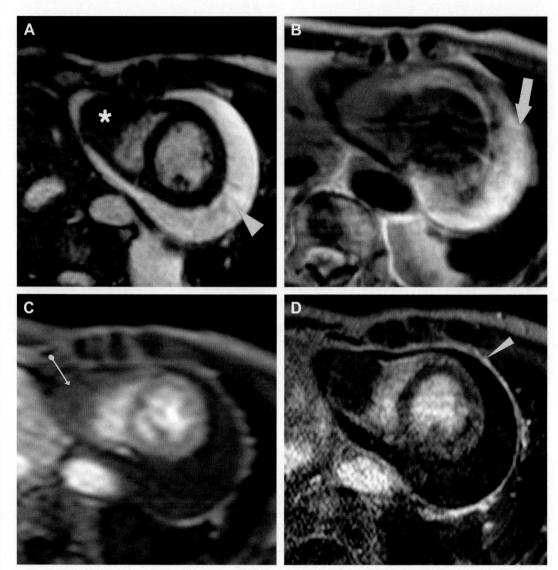

Fig. 8. An 80-year-old man with weight loss and fatigue. Cardiac MR with short-axis images using (A) SSFP, (B) T1W, (C) early perfusion, and (D) LGE sequences. A large mass is evident infiltrating into the acute margin of the right ventricle (*asterisk*). A large pericardial effusion has increased signal on SSFP sequence, which has properties of T2-weighting (*broad arrowhead*). Increased signal within the pericardial effusion is also incidentally noted on T1 sequences (*thick arrow*). Typically fluid is dark on T1 sequences. In this case, the increased signal suggests that the fluid contains proteinaceous or hemorrhagic components, which would be bright on T1 sequences. Mild decreased early enhancement of the mass is noted on first pass perfusion (*thin arrow*). Enhancement of the pericardium is noted on the LGE sequences consistent with pericardial inflammation (*thin arrowhead*), whereas the mass itself remains similar in signal to the myocardium.

recent series of 14 PCLs included 6 DLBCLs, 4 Burkitt lymphomas, 2 PELs, and one each of large cell anaplastic and follicular lymphoma.[25] In this series, the most common site was the right atrium.[25]

DLBCL results in a monomorphous population of lymphoid cells that express B-cell antigens, reflecting either germinal center or nongerminal center lineage by immunohistochemical stains or flow cytometry. The establishment of B-cell lineage requires demonstration of B-cell markers, such as CD19, CD20, CD22, CD79a, or PAX-5. The most common type of cardiac DLBCL is the classic type. Variants of DLBCL that have been described in the heart include DLBCL associated with chronic inflammation

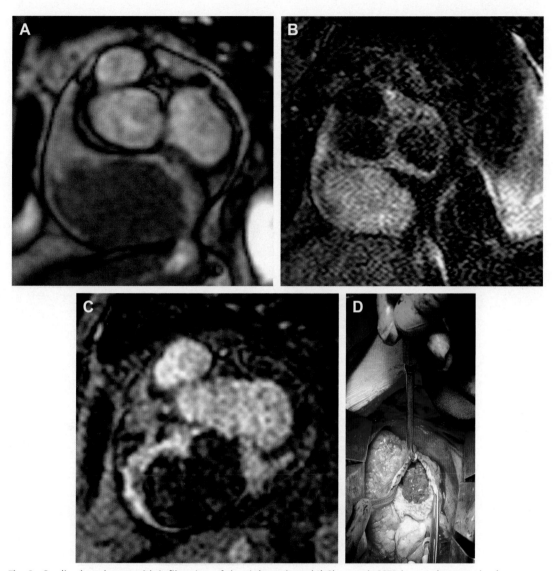

Fig. 9. Cardiac lymphoma with infiltration of the right atrium. (*A*) Short-axis SSFP image shows an isodense mass infiltrating the right atrium with significant intracavitary extension. (*B*) T2W images reveal the mass to be isodense relative to the myocardium. (*C*) Inversion recovery sequence assessing LGE exhibits nulling of the mass at the same inversion time as myocardial nulling. (*D*) Intraoperative view of opened right atrium shows a multilobulated pink mass within the chamber representing cardiac lymphoma.

and PEL. The former include lymphomas arising in association with prosthetic valves and synthetic grafts, which are often EBV-positive.[71–74] PEL is a distinct type of lymphoma arising in association with HHV-8 infection in immunocompromised patients. The pericardium is an unusual site for PEL.[11,48,75–78] Histologically, effusion lymphomas bridge features of large-cell immunoblastic and anaplastic large-cell lymphoma. Most of these cases comprise a unique subgroup of B-cell lymphoma, but T-cell and natural killer cell immunophenotypes are described.[79]

Endemic-type Burkitt lymphoma (occurring in children with EBV infection) has not been reported in the heart, but sporadic and immunodeficiency-related Burkitt lymphoma may occur within the pericardium. Burkitt lymphoma is defined by morphologic features and the expression of pan-B-cell antigens, including CD19, CD20, CD22, and CD79a, and coexpression of CD10, Bcl-6, and CD43. The cells of

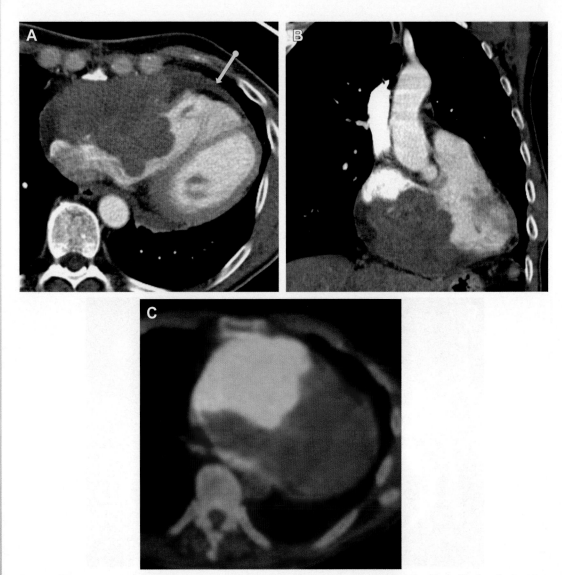

Fig. 10. A 58-year-old patient with a 3-month history of increasing dyspnea and pericardial effusion detected on recent echocardiography. (*A, B*) Contrast-enhanced axial CT and coronal multiplanar reformatted images demonstrate a large homogeneous mass broadly infiltrating the right heart border and extending into right atrial and ventricular chambers. Note associated small pericardial effusion (*arrow*). (*C*) FDG-PET/CT confirms elevated metabolic activity within the mass and absence of activity elsewhere in the body.

Box 2
Radiologic differential diagnosis
Lung cancer with secondary cardiac involvement
Metastatic melanoma (or other metastases)
Benign primary cardiac neoplasms (eg, atypical atrial myxoma)
Angiosarcoma or other undifferentiated sarcoma
Metastatic pericardial effusion

classic Burkitt morphology are relatively small with multiple small chromocenters and dark blue cytoplasm; plasmacytoid features are common in immunodeficiency-related Burkitt lymphoma, and there can be moderate pleomorphism in atypical Burkitt lymphoma. Unlike follicular lymphomas, there is lack of expression of CD5, CD23, and Bcl-2. Diagnosis is often corroborated by characteristic gene translocations, specifically between the *c-myc* gene and the *IgH* gene [t(8;14)] or between c-*myc* and the gene for either

Table 3
Imaging findings

Feature	CT	MR Imaging
Infiltrative intramural mass with propensity for invasion of right cardiac chambers	Isodense to myocardium	T1W: isointense to myocardium T2W: isointense to mildly hyperintense SSFP: isointense to myocardium
Contrast enhancement	Poor	Early: variable Delayed: similar to myocardium
Necrosis	Less likely to demonstrate central necrosis that cardiac sarcomas	
Pericardium	Pericardial implants or thickening with pericardial effusion common	
Vena cava	Obstruction of superior or inferior vena cava possible with extreme cases causing SVC syndrome or lower extremity edema	
Valves	May encroach on valvular structure but not typically a direct cause of valvular abnormality	
Metabolic activity (nuclear medicine imaging)	Correlation of findings from CT or MR imaging with complementary physiologic information from nuclear medicine increases diagnostic accuracy • Uptake with Gallium-67 can be nonspecific • FDG-PET is useful in evaluating intracardiac and extracardiac involvement as well as assessing response to chemotherapy	

Adapted from Jeudy J, Kirsch J, Tavora F, et al. From the radiologic pathology archives: cardiac lymphoma: radiologic-pathologic correlation. Radiographics 2012;32(5):1369–80; and Burke A, Tavora F. Hematologic tumors of the heart and pericardium. In: Burke A, Tavora F, Maleszewski J, et al, editors. Tumors of the heart and great vessels, AFIP Atlas of Tumor Pathology. Series 4. vol. 22. Annapolis Junction (MD): American Registry of Pathology; 2015. p. 337–52.

the κ or λ light chain [t(2;8) or t(8;22), respectively].

In addition to effusion lymphoma, other types of cardiac lymphomas may occur in immunocompromised patients, including patients with HIV-AIDS or allografts.[8,67,80–82] Cardiac lymphomas comprise less than 5% of all lymphomas arising in patients with AIDS and organ transplants. Diffuse large-cell lymphomas, plasmacytoid (plasmablastic) or immunoblastic lymphoma, and low-grade B-cell lymphomas are the most common histologic types. A histologic progression from a polyclonal, polymorphous infiltrate to a monoclonal, monomorphous high-grade cardiac lymphoma has been demonstrated in HIV patients analogous to posttransplant lymphoproliferative disease in solid organ transplant patients.[83]

The incidence of secondary cardiac lymphoma in patients with B-cell lymphoma ranges from 9% to 20%.[84] The heart may also be secondarily involved in Hodgkin disease[85] and T-cell lymphomas.[86] There may be direct extension from mediastinal lymphoma, retrograde lymphatic spread in lymphatics along the coronary arteries and in the epicardium, and hematogenous spread. Hematogenous spread is characterized by interstitial and epicardial masses that resemble abscesses and is typical of low-grade and intermediate follicular lymphomas. Both Hodgkin lymphomas and high-grade non-Hodgkin lymphomas are more likely to spread to the heart by direct extension or lymphatic routes.[87]

TREATMENT AND PROGNOSIS

Management of cardiac lymphoma is varied. Medical literature presents a myriad of treatment combinations including modalities of chemotherapy, radiotherapy, surgery, and even autologous stem cell transplantation.[1,70,88] Surgery is usually palliative and used for tumor debulking. Investigators propose that PCL should be considered a systemic disease and that treatment should always include chemotherapy.[6]

The main chemotherapeutic regimen for cardiac lymphoma includes anthracycline-containing agents, including cyclophosphamide, doxorubicin + vincristine + prednisone

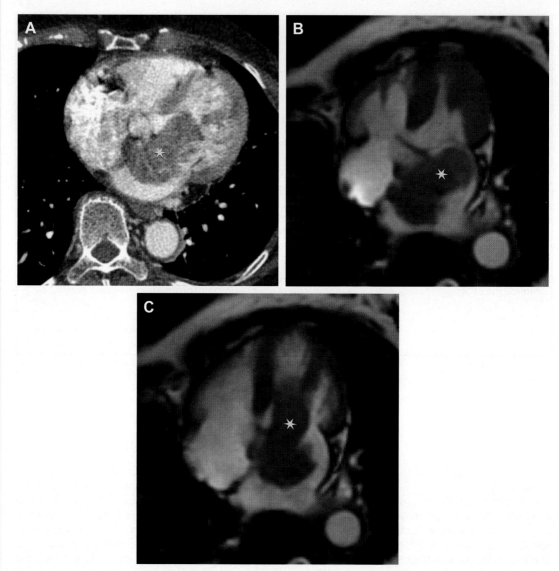

Fig. 11. A 78-year-old patient with left atrial mass. (*A*) Contrast-enhanced axial cardiac CT shows a large left atrial mass (star) arising from the interatrial septum, extending into the left atrium and further prolapsing through the mitral valve into the left ventricle. (*B, C*) Horizontal long-axis SSFP images during systole and diastole demonstrate dynamic movement of the mass (star) without evidence of valve obstruction. Although cardiac myxoma was the primary consideration by imaging criteria, immunohistochemistry revealed the mass to be a PCL (DLBCL).

(CHOP).[3] In one review, patients treated with CHOP survived for up to 18 months, whereas those treated with the BACOP protocol (bleomycin + doxorubicin + cyclophosphamide + vincristine + prednisone) survived for up to 49 months. Patients who underwent surgical resection survived for more than 18 months and with radiotherapy for up to 15 months.[89] The monoclonal CD20 antibody (Rituximab) has been found to induce regression in B-cell non-Hodgkin lymphomas in CD20-positive patients and has shown potential to increase the overall survival rate when added to the CHOP protocol.[90,91]

There are known complications specifically related to the treatment of cardiac lymphoma, including cardiotoxic effects of certain chemotherapeutics and the sequelae of radiation therapy. The potential for cardiac rupture following chemotherapy and the risk for emboli originating from a fragile tumor are of special concern.[92,93] Some investigators recommend a 50% dose reduction of

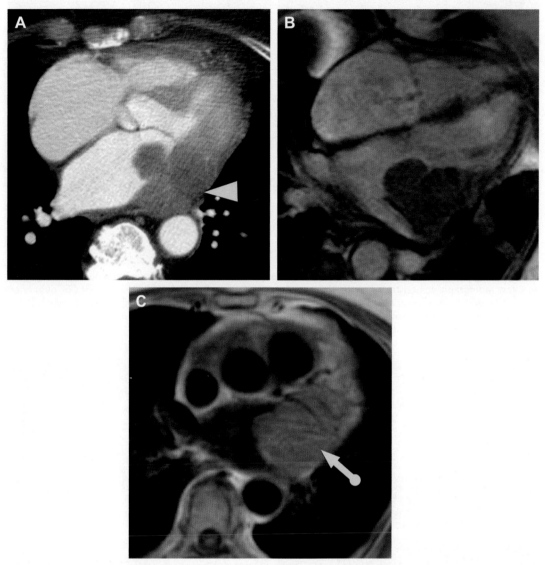

Fig. 12. An 86-year-old patient with a history of renal cell carcinoma. (*A*) Contrast-enhanced axial CT image demonstrates a large mass centered in the left posterior atrioventricular groove with intracavitary extension into left atrium and involvement of left inferior pulmonary vein (*arrowhead*). (*B, C*) Horizontal long-axis SSFP and T1W MR images show the mass to be isointense to myocardium (*arrow*). Given the location and features of vascular invasion, a primary sarcoma was favored, but immunohistochemistry analysis of the tissue revealed DLBCL. No other sites of lymphomatous involvement were identified.

cyclophosphamide and adriamycin to be administered during the initial course, in order to avoid the risk of sudden death following rapid tumor regression.[47]

The prognosis for patients with either primary or secondary cardiac lymphoma is usually poor. A recent analysis of PCL and treatment outcome patterns (including a cohort of 128 patients treated with chemotherapy, surgery, radiation, or chemotherapy/radiation combined) demonstrated a median overall survival of approximately 12 months.[6] Initial nonspecific signs and symptoms, rapid evolution of cardiac involvement, and late diagnosis are major factors affecting the outcome.[7,80,90,94] Four key adverse prognostic factors are being immunocompromised, the presence of extracardiac disease, left ventricular involvement, and absence of arrhythmia. The last of these factors is surprising, but investigators suggest that the presence of arrhythmia may prompt earlier clinical presentation, leading to more timely treatment of the disease.[6]

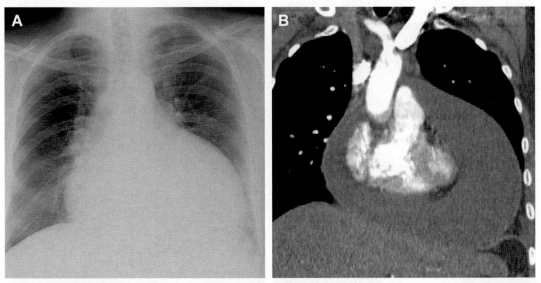

Fig. 13. A 48-year-old man with a history of HIV and Kaposi sarcoma presented with a large pericardial effusion. (*A*) Chest radiograph demonstrates marked enlargement of the cardiac silhouette. No evidence of pulmonary vascular congestion or pleural effusion is observed. (*B*) Coronal MPR from contrast-enhanced CT reveals that a large pericardial effusion explains the chest radiograph findings. Cytopathologic evaluation of aspirated pericardial fluid confirmed markers of HHV-8 consistent with PEL.

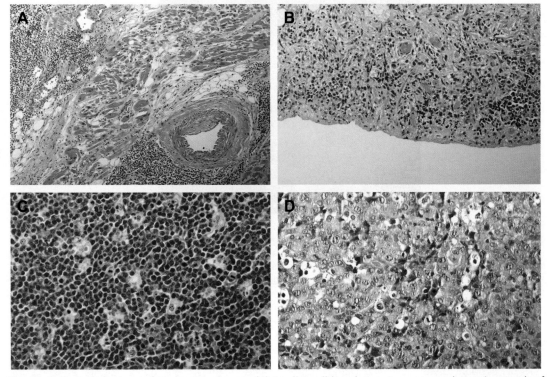

Fig. 14. Pathologic features of cardiac lymphomas. (*A*) Small B-cell lymphoma. Low-power photomicrograph of myocardium shows diffuse infiltrates of small lymphocytes with myocytes and intracardiac adipose tissue. (*B*) PEL. Medium-power photomicrograph of the pericardial surface shows tumor cells with pleomorphism, irregular nuclei, and abundant cytoplasm. (*C*) Burkitt lymphoma. High-power photomicrograph shows medium-sized tumor cells with a diffuse monotonous pattern. There are numerous mitotic figures. Scattered macrophages produce a "starry sky" pattern. (*D*) DLBCL. Photomicrograph shows very large round to oval cells with bizarre pleomorphic nuclei that grow in a cohesive pattern, thus mimicking carcinoma. (*Reprinted from* Jeudy J, Kirsch J, Tavora F, et al. From the radiologic pathology archives: cardiac lymphoma: radiologic-pathologic correlation. Radiographics 2012;32(5):1377; with permission.)

SUMMARY

PCL is rare and accounts for less than 2% of primary cardiac tumors (**Box 3**). On the other hand, secondary cardiac involvement is reported in 25% of patients with disseminated nodal lymphoma. Cardiac lymphomas are characteristically a subtype of non-Hodgkin lymphoma, of B-cell lineage, and most often DLBCL. PCL usually occurs in older immunocompetent men, although subtypes arise in immunocompromised patients. These subtypes include EBV-associated PTLD and PEL. Cardiac lymphoma manifests as singular or multiple intramural masses with infiltrative margins and a strong predilection for the right heart. Pericardial involvement with effusion is typical. Clinical signs and symptoms reveal its cardiac origin and include dysrhythmias, congestive heart failure, pericardial effusion, cardiac tamponade, and superior vena caval syndrome.

Multimodality imaging optimizes the diagnostic evaluation. Echocardiography is often the initial imaging modality, but CT and MR imaging provide superior soft tissue contrast and anatomic information. Nuclear medicine imaging (18F-FDG-PET/CT) may assist in therapeutic management. Diagnosis is ultimately confirmed by direct tissue biopsy or pericardial fluid cytology. Unlike other cardiac tumors, which often require surgical resection, treatment of cardiac lymphoma comprises anthracycline-based chemotherapy with anti-CD20 (Rituximab), in some cases combined with radiation therapy. Overall prognosis remains poor.

Box 3
Cardiac lymphoma: clinical pearls

Primary cardiac lymphoma is rare, whereas secondary involvement of the heart is present in 25% of patients with disseminated lymphoma

Almost all cardiac lymphomas are B-cell origin (usually diffuse large B-cell lymphoma)

Usually arise in immunocompetent older adults (M > F, mean age 60 years)

Subsets occur in immunocompromised patients, HIV-positive, or allograft recipients (EBV-associated lymphoproliferative disorders; PEL)

Complications include conduction disturbances, congestive heart failure, pericardial effusion, cardiac tamponade, vena caval obstruction, embolic phenomena, coronary arterial infiltration

Tumor staging includes direct tissue sampling along with bone marrow biopsies, whole body CT, and/or MR imaging, nuclear medicine PET scanning

---

REFERENCES

1. Burke A, Tavora F. Hematologic tumors of the heart and pericardium. In: Burke A, Tavora F, Maleszewski J, et al, editors. Tumors of the heart and great vessels. Annapolis Junction (MD): American Registry of Pathology; 2015. p. 337–52.
2. Gowda RM, Khan IA. Clinical perspectives of primary cardiac lymphoma. Angiology 2003;54(5): 599–604.
3. Travis WD, Brambilla E, Burke AP, et al. WHO classification of tumours of the lung, pleura, thymus and heart. 4th edition. Lyon (France): International Agency for Research on Cancer (IARC); 2015.
4. Burke A, Tavora F, Maleszewski M, et al. Tumors of the heart and great vessels. AFIP Atlas of Tumor Pathology, 4th series, Vol 22. Silver Spring (MD): American Registry of Pathology; 2015.
5. Burke A, Jeudy J Jr, Virmani R. Cardiac tumours: an update: cardiac tumours. Heart 2008;94(1):117–23.
6. Petrich A, Cho S, Billett H. Primary cardiac lymphoma: an analysis of presentation, treatment and outcome patterns. Cancer 2011;117:581–9.
7. Chalabreysse L, Berger F, Loire R, et al. Primary cardiac lymphoma in immunocompetent patients: a report of three cases and review of the literature. Virchows Arch 2002;441(5):456–61.
8. Holladay AO, Siegel RJ, Schwartz DA. Cardiac malignant lymphoma in acquired immune deficiency syndrome. Cancer 1992;70(8):2203–7.
9. Kaplan LD. HIV-associated lymphoma. Best Pract Res Clin Haematol 2012;25(1):101–17.
10. Carter BW, Wu CC, Khorashadi L, et al. Multimodality imaging of cardiothoracic lymphoma. Eur J Radiol 2014;83(8):1470–82.
11. Chen Y-B, Rahemtullah A, Hochberg E. Primary effusion lymphoma. Oncologist 2007;12:569–76.
12. Simonelli C, Spina M, Cinelli R, et al. Clinical features and outcome of primary effusion lymphoma in HIV-infected patients: a single-institution study. J Clin Oncol 2003;21(21):3948–54.
13. Curtsinger CR, Wilson MJ, Yoneda K. Primary cardiac lymphoma. Cancer 1989;64(2):521–5.
14. Miguel CE, Bestetti RB. Primary cardiac lymphoma. Int J Cardiol 2011;149(3):358–63.
15. Tai CJ, Wang WS, Chung MT, et al. Complete atrioventricular block as a major clinical presentation of the primary cardiac lymphoma: a case report. Jpn J Clin Oncol 2001;31(5):217–20.
16. Chinen K, Izumo T. Cardiac involvement by malignant lymphoma: a clinicopathologic study of 25 autopsy cases based on the WHO classification. Ann Hematol 2005;84(8):498–505.
17. Patel J, Melly L, Sheppard MN. Primary cardiac lymphoma: B- and T-cell cases at a specialist UK centre. Ann Oncol 2010;21(5):1041–5.

18. Perez Baztarrica G, Nieva N, Gariglio L, et al. Images in cardiovascular medicine. Primary cardiac lymphoma: a rare case of pulmonary tumor embolism. Circulation 2010;121(20):2249–50.

19. Habertheuer A, Ehrlich M, Wiedemann D, et al. A rare case of primary cardiac B cell lymphoma. J Cardiothorac Surg 2014;9:14.

20. Ryu SJ, Choi BW, Choe KO. CT and MR findings of primary cardiac lymphoma: report upon 2 cases and review. Yonsei Med J 2001;42(4):451–6.

21. Kim EY, Choe YH, Sung K, et al. Multidetector CT and MR imaging of cardiac tumors. Korean J Radiol 2009;10(2):164–75.

22. Buckley O, Madan R, Kwong R, et al. Cardiac masses, part 1: imaging strategies and technical considerations. AJR Am J Roentgenol 2011;197(5):W837–41.

23. Ceresoli GL, Ferreri AJM, Bucci E, et al. Primary cardiac lymphoma in immunocompetent patients: diagnostic and therapeutic management. Cancer 1997; 80(8):1497–506.

24. Dorsay TA, Ho VB, Rovira MJ, et al. Primary cardiac lymphoma: CT and MR findings. J Comput Assist Tomogr 1993;17(6):978–81.

25. Jeudy J, Kirsch J, Tavora F, et al. From the radiologic pathology archives: cardiac lymphoma: radiologic-pathologic correlation. Radiographics 2012;32(5): 1369–80.

26. Abdullah HN, Nowalid WK. Infiltrative cardiac lymphoma with tricuspid valve involvement in a young man. World J Cardiol 2014;6(2):77–80.

27. Zlotchenko G, Futuri S, Dillon E, et al. A rare case of lymphoma involving the tricuspid valve. J Cardiovasc Comput Tomogr 2013;7(3):207–9.

28. Gosev I, Siric F, Gasparovic H, et al. Surgical treatment of a primary cardiac lymphoma presenting with tamponade physiology. J Card Surg 2006; 21(4):414–6.

29. Hwang MH, Brown A, Piao ZE, et al. Cardiac lymphoma associated with superior vena caval syndrome and cardiac tamponade: case history. Angiology 1990;41(4):328–32.

30. Nagamine K, Noda H. Two cases of primary cardiac lymphoma presenting with pericardial effusion and cardiac tamponade. Jpn Circ J 1990;54(9): 1158–64.

31. Wilhite DB, Quigley RL. Occult cardiac lymphoma presenting with cardiac tamponade. Tex Heart Inst J 2003;30(1):62–4.

32. O'Donnell DH, Abbara S, Chaithiraphan V, et al. Cardiac tumors: optimal cardiac MR sequences and spectrum of imaging appearances. Am J Roentgenol 2009;193(2):377–87.

33. Kramer CM, Barkhausen J, Flamm SD, Society for Cardiovascular Magnetic Resonance, et al. Standardized cardiovascular magnetic resonance (CMR) protocols 2013 update. J Cardiovasc Magn Reson 2013;15(1):91.

34. Mitchell DG, Burk DL Jr, Vinitski S, et al. The biophysical basis of tissue contrast in extracranial MR imaging. AJR Am J Roentgenol 1987;149(4): 831–7.

35. Johnson BA, Fram EK, Johnson PC, et al. The variable MR appearance of primary lymphoma of the central nervous system: comparison with histopathologic features. AJNR Am J Neuroradiol 1997; 18(3):563–72.

36. Araoz PA, Eklund HE, Welch TJ, et al. CT and MR imaging of primary cardiac malignancies. Radiographics 1999;19(6):1421–34.

37. Restrepo CS, Largoza A, Lemos DF, et al. CT and MR imaging findings of malignant cardiac tumors. Curr Probl Diagn Radiol 2005;34(1):1–11.

38. Partovi S, Karimi S, Lyo JK, et al. Multimodality imaging of primary CNS lymphoma in immunocompetent patients. Br J Radiol 2014;87(1036):20130684.

39. Khuddus MA, Schmalfuss CM, Aranda JM, et al. Magnetic resonance imaging of primary cardiac lymphoma. Clin Cardiol 2007;30(3):144–5.

40. Grizzard JD, Ang GB. Magnetic resonance imaging of pericardial disease and cardiac masses. Magn Reson Imaging Clin N Am 2007;15(4):579–607, vi.

41. Weinsaft JW, Kim HW, Shah DJ, et al. Detection of left ventricular thrombus by delayed-enhancement cardiovascular magnetic resonance prevalence and markers in patients with systolic dysfunction. J Am Coll Cardiol 2008;52(2):148–57.

42. Hamada S, Nishimura T, Hayashida K, et al. Intracardiac malignant lymphoma detected by gallium-67 citrate and thallium-201 chloride. J Nucl Med 1988; 29(11):1868–70.

43. Okada M, Sato N, Ishii K, et al. FDG PET/CT versus CT, MR imaging, and 67Ga scintigraphy in the post-therapy evaluation of malignant lymphoma. Radiographics 2010;30(4):939–57.

44. Raanani P, Shasha Y, Perry C, et al. Is CT scan still necessary for staging in Hodgkin and non-Hodgkin lymphoma patients in the PET/CT era? Ann Oncol 2006;17(1):117–22.

45. Montiel V, Maziers N, Dereme T. Primary cardiac lymphoma and complete atrio-ventricular block: case report and review of the literature. Acta Cardiol 2007;62(1):55–8.

46. Freudenberg LS, Antoch G, Schutt P, et al. FDG-PET/CT in re-staging of patients with lymphoma. Eur J Nucl Med Mol Imaging 2004;31(3):325–9.

47. Dawson MA, Mariani J, Taylor A, et al. The successful treatment of primary cardiac lymphoma with a dose-dense schedule of rituximab plus CHOP. Ann Oncol 2006;17(1):176–7.

48. Bhargava P, Glass E, Brown J, et al. FDG PET in primary effusion lymphoma (PEL) of the pericardium. Clin Nucl Med 2006;31(1):18–9.

49. Engelen MA, Bruch C, Buerger H, et al. Pericarditis constrictiva and high-degree atrioventricular block

as a first manifestation of a cardiac B-cell lymphoma. J Am Soc Echocardiogr 2005;18(6):694.

50. Thakrar A, Farag A, Lytwyn M, et al. Multimodality cardiac imaging for the noninvasive characterization of intracardiac neoplasms. Int J Cardiol 2009;132(2): e74–6.

51. Mato AR, Morgans AK, Roullet MR, et al. Primary cardiac lymphoma: utility of multimodality imaging in diagnosis and management. Cancer Biol Ther 2007;6(12):1867–70.

52. Burke AP, Tavora F. Cardiac lymphoma and metastatic tumors to the heart. In: Burke AP, Tavora F, editors. Practical cardiovascular pathology. Philadelphia: Lippincott Williams & Wilkins; 2010. p. 409–506.

53. Tamura A, Matsubara O, Yoshimura N, et al. Cardiac metastasis of lung cancer. A study of metastatic pathways and clinical manifestations. Cancer 1992;70(2):437–42.

54. Sosvińska-Mielcarek K, Senkus-Konefka E, Jassem J, et al. Cardiac involvement at presentation of non–small-cell lung cancer. J Clin Oncol 2008;26(6): 1010–1.

55. Chiles C, Woodard PK, Gutierrez FR, et al. Metastatic involvement of the heart and pericardium: CT and MR imaging. Radiographics 2001;21(2):439–49.

56. Roberts WC. Primary and secondary neoplasms of the heart. Am J Cardiol 1997;80(5):671–82.

57. Tesolin M, Lapierre C, Oligny L, et al. Cardiac metastases from melanoma. Radiographics 2005;25(1): 249–53.

58. Hammoudeh AJ, Chaaban F, Watson RM, et al. Transesophageal echocardiography-guided transvenous endomyocardial biopsy used to diagnose primary cardiac angiosarcoma. Cathet Cardiovasc Diagn 1996;37(3):347–9.

59. Heenan S, Ignotus P, Cox I, et al. Case report: percutaneous biopsy of a right atrial angiosarcoma under ultrasound guidance. Clin Radiol 1996;51(8): 591–2.

60. Park SM, Kang WC, Park CH, et al. Rapidly growing angiosarcoma of the pericardium presenting as hemorrhagic pericardial effusion. Int J Cardiol 2008;130(1):109–12.

61. Grebenc ML, Rosado de Christenson ML, Burke AP, et al. Primary cardiac and pericardial neoplasms: radiologic-pathologic correlation. Radiographics 2000;20(4):1073–103 [quiz: 1110–1, 1112].

62. Rolla G, Calligaris-Cappio F, Burke A. Tumors of the heart: cardiac lymphomas. In: Travis WD, World Health Organization, International Agency for Research on Cancer, International Academy of Pathology, editors. Pathology and genetics of tumors of the lung, pleura, thymus and heart. Lyon (France): IARC Press; 2004.

63. Best AK, Dobson RL, Ahmad AR. Best cases from the AFIP: cardiac angiosarcoma. Radiographics 2003;23 Spec No:S141–5.

64. Yahata S, Endo T, Honma H, et al. Sunray appearance on enhanced magnetic resonance image of cardiac angiosarcoma with pericardial obliteration. Am Heart J 1994;127(2):468–71.

65. Colin GC, Symons R, Dymarkowski S, et al. Value of CMR to differentiate cardiac angiosarcoma from cardiac lymphoma. JACC Cardiovasc Imaging 2015; 8(6):744–6.

66. Roberts WC, Glancy DL, DeVita VT Jr. Heart in malignant lymphoma (Hodgkin's disease, lymphosarcoma, reticulum cell sarcoma and mycosis fungoides). A study of 196 autopsy cases. Am J Cardiol 1968;22(1):85–107.

67. Nart D, Nalbantgil S, Yagdi T, et al. Primary cardiac lymphoma in a heart transplant recipient. Transplant Proc 2005;37(2):1362–4.

68. Ying AJ, Myerowitz PD Jr, Marsh WL. Posttransplantation lymphoproliferative disorder in cardiac transplant allografts. Ann Thorac Surg 1997;64(6): 1822–4.

69. Gill PS, Chandraratna PA, Meyer PR, et al. Malignant lymphoma: cardiac involvement at initial presentation. J Clin Oncol 1987;5(2):216–24.

70. Ikeda H, Nakamura S, Nishimaki H, et al. Primary lymphoma of the heart: case report and literature review. Pathol Int 2004;54(3):187–95.

71. Miller DV, Firchau DJ, McClure RF, et al. Epstein-Barr virus-associated diffuse large B-cell lymphoma arising on cardiac prostheses. Am J Surg Pathol 2010;34(3):377–84.

72. Albat B, Messner-Pellenc P, Thevenet A. Surgical treatment for primary lymphoma of the heart simulating prosthetic mitral valve thrombosis. J Thorac Cardiovasc Surg 1994;108(1):188–9.

73. Bagwan IN, Desai S, Wotherspoon A, et al. Unusual presentation of primary cardiac lymphoma. Interact Cardiovasc Thorac Surg 2009;9(1):127–9.

74. Durrleman NM, El-Hamamsy I, Demaria RG, et al. Cardiac lymphoma following mitral valve replacement. Ann Thorac Surg 2005;79(3):1040–2.

75. Inoue Y, Tsukasaki K, Nagai K, et al. Durable remission by sobuzoxane in an HIV-seronegative patient with human herpesvirus 8-negative primary effusion lymphoma. Int J Hematol 2004;79(3):271–5.

76. Kishimoto K, Kitamura T, Hirayama Y, et al. Cytologic and immunocytochemical features of EBV negative primary effusion lymphoma: report on seven Japanese cases. Diagn Cytopathol 2009;37(4):293–8.

77. Nakakuki T, Masuoka H, Ishikura K, et al. A case of primary cardiac lymphoma located in the pericardial effusion. Heart Vessels 2004;19(4):199–202.

78. Won J-H, Han S-H, Bae S-B, et al. Successful eradication of relapsed primary effusion lymphoma with high-dose chemotherapy and autologous stem cell transplantation in a patient seronegative for human immunodeficiency virus. Int J Hematol 2006;83(4): 328–30.

79. Das DK. Serous effusions in malignant lymphomas: a review. Diagn Cytopathol 2006;34(5):335–47.

80. Sanna P, Bertoni F, Zucca E, et al. Cardiac involvement in HIV-related non-Hodgkin's lymphoma: a case report and short review of the literature. Ann Hematol 1998;77(1–2):75–8.

81. Khan NUA, Ahmed S, Wagner P, et al. Cardiac involvement in non-Hodgkin's lymphoma: with and without HIV infection. Int J Cardiovasc Imaging 2004 Dec;20(6):477–81.

82. Barbaro G, Di Lorenzo G, Grisorio B, et al. Cardiac involvement in the acquired immunodeficiency syndrome: a multicenter clinical-pathological study. Gruppo Italiano per lo Studio Cardiologico dei pazienti affetti da AIDS Investigators. AIDS Res Hum Retroviruses 1998;14(12):1071–7.

83. Guarner J, Brynes RK, Chan WC, et al. Primary non-Hodgkin's lymphoma of the heart in two patients with the acquired immunodeficiency syndrome. Arch Pathol Lab Med 1987;111(3):254–6.

84. O'Mahony D, Peikarz RL, Bandettini WP, et al. Cardiac involvement with lymphoma: a review of the literature. Clin Lymphoma Myeloma 2008;8(4): 249–52.

85. Retter A, Ardeshna KM, O'Driscoll A. Cardiac tamponade in Hodgkin lymphoma. Br J Haematol 2007;138(1):2.

86. Iemura A, Yano H, Kojiro M, et al. Massive cardiac involvement of adult T-cell leukemia/lymphoma. An autopsy case. Arch Pathol Lab Med 1991;115(10): 1052–4.

87. McDonnell PJ, Mann RB, Bulkley BH. Involvement of the heart by malignant lymphoma: a clinicopathologic study. Cancer 1982;49(5):944–51.

88. Potenza L, Luppi M, Morselli M, et al. Cardiac involvement in malignancies. Case 2. Right ventricular lesion as presenting feature of acute promyelocytic leukemia. J Clin Oncol 2004;22(13): 2742–4.

89. Hsueh S-C, Chung M-T, Fang R, et al. Primary cardiac lymphoma. J Chin Med Assoc 2006;69(4): 169–74.

90. Morillas P, Quiles J, Nuñez D, et al. Complete regression of cardiac non-Hodgkin lymphoma. Int J Cardiol 2006;106(3):426–7.

91. Takenaka S, Mitsudo K, Inoue K, et al. Successful treatment of primary cardiac lymphoma with atrioventricular nodal block. Int Heart J 2005;46(5): 927–31.

92. Molajo AO, McWilliam L, Ward C, et al. Cardiac lymphoma: an unusual case of myocardial perforation–clinical, echocardiographic, haemodynamic and pathological features. Eur Heart J 1987;8(5): 549–52.

93. Kosugi M, Ono T, Yamaguchi H, et al. Successful treatment of primary cardiac lymphoma and pulmonary tumor embolism with chemotherapy. Int J Cardiol 2006;111(1):172–3.

94. Rolla G, Bertero MT, Pastena G, et al. Primary lymphoma of the heart. A case report and review of the literature. Leuk Res 2002;26(1):117–20.

Extranodal Lymphoma of the Breast

Brandi T. Nicholson, MD[a],*, Rahat M. Bhatti, MD[b], Leonard Glassman, MD[c]

KEYWORDS

- Extranodal lymphoma • Breast • Primary breast lymphoma • Secondary breast lymphoma
- B-cell lymphoma

KEY POINTS

- Extranodal lymphoma (ENL) of the breast is an uncommon disease and typically presents in middle-aged women as a unilateral palpable breast mass.
- B-cell lymphoma is the most common ENL of the breast.
- Imaging is unable to distinguish lymphoma from breast cancer, which is more common; therefore, biopsy is done to establish the diagnosis.

INTRODUCTION

The breast is an uncommon location for ENL to present, occurring in only 2% of all localized ENLs,[1] and ENL encompasses fewer than 0.5% of all breast malignancies.[2] Overall leukemia and lymphoma, however, are the most common sources of extramammary cancer involving the breast.[3,4] Breast lymphoma (BL) typically presents in 1 of 2 clinical scenarios. These include primary BL (PBL) and secondary involvement of breast tissue by a systemic lymphoma/leukemia, or secondary BL (SBL).[5,6] The term PBL is used when a patient has a malignant lymphoma primarily occurring in the breast without previous known lymphoma.[7] A vast majority of lymphomas involving the breast are seen in women; however, rarely, cases have occurred in men.[8–12]

The origins of BL are not completely understood. It has been postulated that the breast can act as a mucosal immune system site with development of lymphoid tissue associated with autoimmune mechanisms or other inciting events, or in general terms the breast may behave as a mucosal-associated lymphoid tissue.[4,13] Some studies have shown higher rates of BL in patients with autoimmune diseases, in particular Sjögren syndrome and systemic lupus erythematosus.[14,15] Given that not all BLs are associated with autoimmune disease, however, other mechanisms must exist. Some have postulated that BL may arise from intraparenchymal lymphatics or intramammary lymph nodes.[13]

SBL is more common than PBL. When PBL occurs, the most common type is diffuse large B-cell lymphoma (DLBCL). DLBCL typically occurs in the 5th or 6th decade with a unilateral, solitary, palpable mass, indistinguishable from a breast cancer.[2,9,16–18] Fig. 1 shows the common imaging appearance and various pathology of B-cell lymphoma. These patients uncommonly have the systemic symptoms of mastalgia or B symptoms (fever, chills, and night sweats); therefore, diagnosis is usually only obtained after a breast

Disclosures: Siemens; Readers study for tomosynthesis Food and Drug Administration submission, compensated for time (B.T. Nicholson). None (R. Bhatti and L. Glassman).
[a] Department of Radiology & Medical Imaging, University of Virginia, Charlottesville, VA 22908, USA; [b] Department of Pathology, University of Virginia, Charlottesville, VA 22908, USA; [c] Washington Radiology Associates PC, Washington, DC 20037, USA
* Corresponding author.
E-mail address: bte6v@virginia.edu

Radiol Clin N Am 54 (2016) 711–726
http://dx.doi.org/10.1016/j.rcl.2016.03.005
0033-8389/16/$ – see front matter © 2016 Elsevier Inc. All rights reserved.

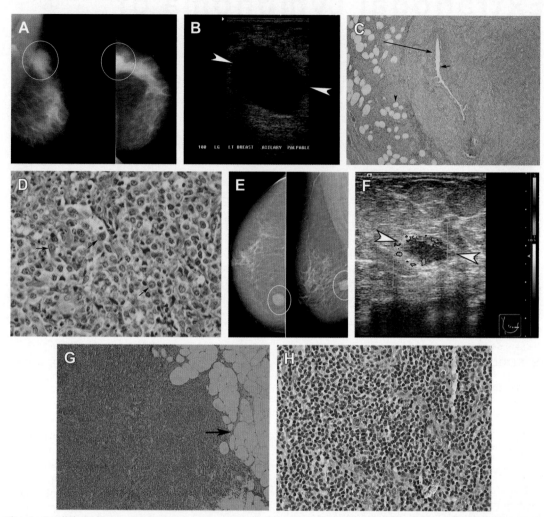

Fig. 1. B-cell lymphoma, both (*A–D*) high-grade (DLBCL) and (*E–H*) low-grade tumor types. (*A*) Diagnostic mammogram, mediolateral-oblique (MLO) and cranial-caudal (CC) views, performed for a palpable left breast mass in a middle-aged woman reveals a round, obscured, equal-density mass in the upper outer left breast (*circles*). (*B*) Subsequent ultrasound shows a round, indistinct, hypoechoic solid mass (*arrowheads*). (*C*) Hematoxylin-eosin stain at low power demonstrates sheets of tumor cells (*long arrow*) in close approximation to a duct (*short arrow*) and mammary adipose tissue (*arrowhead*). (*D*) Hematoxylin-eosin stain at high power shows tumor cells that have large, irregular nuclei consistent with a high-grade process (*arrows*). (*E*) A second patient presented with a screening detected oval, circumscribed, equal-density right breast mass (*circles*) on CC and MLO views. (*F*) Ultrasound shows an oval, indistinct, and hypoechoic solid mass with increased vascularity (*arrowheads*). (*G*) Hematoxylin-eosin stain at low power shows sheets of small cells infiltrating fat (*arrow*) with a diffuse growth pattern. (*H*) Hematoxylin-eosin stain at high power shows small cells with a monotonous pattern, consistent with a low-grade process.

biopsy.[19] Less commonly, PBL presents in a pregnant or recently pregnant younger woman as bilateral high-grade malignant lymphoma. This type of PBL, which is commonly a rapidly disseminating Burkitt lymphoma, tends to spread to the central nervous system, ovaries, gastrointestinal tract, or endocrine organs. **Fig. 2** shows the imaging appearance of a more aggressive Burkitt lymphoma.

Given the rarity of BL, it is not usually suspected in the presentation of a palpable breast mass. It is important to secure a diagnosis via biopsy because the treatment of BL is different from that for breast cancer. Surgery may be done; however, the most successful treatment of BL is a combination of chemotherapy and radiotherapy. Outcomes of PBL differ from those for breast cancer. For PBL, the reported 5-year survival rate is 42% to

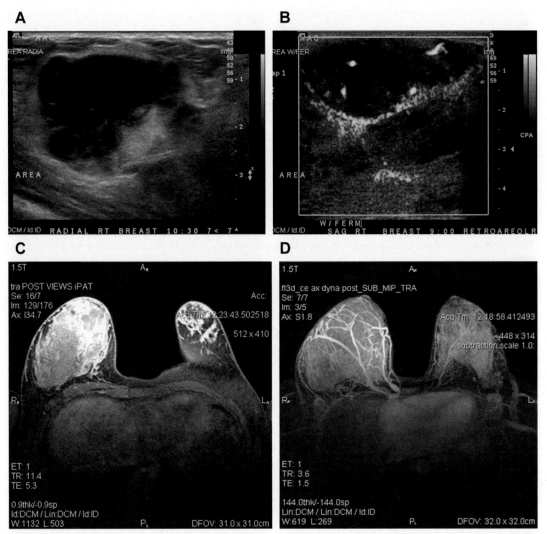

Fig. 2. Burkitt lymphoma. A 27-year-old woman presenting with an enlarging right breast. (*A, B*) Ultrasound was performed due to her young age and shows a large, oval, circumscribed, hypoechoic solid mass with increased vascularity. (*C, D*) Contrast-enhanced breast MR imaging was done during her initial work-up and shows the right breast is replaced by a large enhancing mass with hypervascularity of the entire breast compared with the left. The mass had diffuse increased ^{18}F-FDG uptake on CT-PET, not shown.

83% with a recurrence rate at 15%. This is not as good as in breast cancer, which is 89% and 12% (at 10 years), respectively.[20,21]

NORMAL ANATOMY AND IMAGING TECHNIQUE
Normal Breast Anatomy

The breast begins to develop in the fifth week of fetal life from the primitive milk streaks (milk lines). These milk lines usually regress everywhere except in the chest where the mammary glands begin to form.[22] The ectoderm forms 15 to 20 branching epithelial cords, which extend into the mesoderm, from which the fibrous and fatty tissue develops. The nipple and ductal system are formed in the last 8 weeks of fetal life up to birth. The ducts continue to develop until puberty and, in women, hormones at puberty stimulate the ducts to proliferate and the lobules to form.

A developed breast overlies the chest from the 2nd to 6th ribs, extending from the lateral edge of the sternum to the anterior axillary line laterally. The suspensory ligaments of Cooper support the breast tissue by connecting the breast to the underlying fascia and pectoralis muscle. The normal glandular tissue is made up of ducts, terminal ducts, and acini and is supported by fibrous

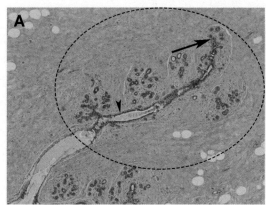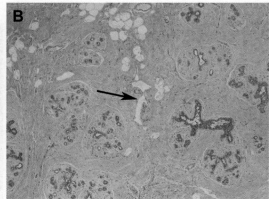

Fig. 3. Hematoxylin-eosin stain of the normal breast tissue. (*A*) Low-power view demonstrates a terminal duct lobular unit (TDLU) (*circle*). The ductal component is seen centrally (*arrowhead*). Several lobular units are present arising from the terminal duct (*arrow*). (*B*) Low-power view shows multiple TDLUs around a lymphatic vessel (*arrow*).

tissue. There are 15 to 20 segments or lobes in the developed breast with each draining at the lactiferous duct into the nipple. **Fig. 3** shows the lobule, the functional unit of the breast, which is made up of the terminal ducts, and acini.[23] The lobules change significantly during the menstrual cycles and after menopause they atrophy and decrease in number.

Abnormalities of the Breast

Most abnormalities of the breast involve the epithelium. There are both ductal and lobular epithelial cells, which can undergo abnormal proliferation with the development of either benign or malignant processes. Breast cancer is the most common malignancy affecting the breast and is divided into ductal and lobular types (both in situ and invasive). Overall, nonepithelial tumors of the breast are rare. Examples include BL, granular cell tumor, stromal cell sarcoma, hemangioma, and angiosarcoma. Metastatic involvement of the breast by extramammary carcinomas is also uncommon.

Breast Lymphatics

Lymphatic capillaries, located in the breast lobules, are tiny, at 10 μm to 50 μm in diameter, with an only 1-cell-layer–thick endothelial lining and a discontinuous basement membrane.[24] Lymph is absorbed into these blind-ending lymphatic capillaries from the interstitial space. The filling of the capillaries and the unidirectional movement, due to the presence of valves, of lymph through the capillaries occur via contractions of smooth muscles in the media and external pressures creating osmotic pressure gradients.[24,25] The lymph then drains into collecting

lymphatic vessels, which drain to a lymph node. The majority of lymphatic drainage (see **Fig. 3**) of the breast begins at the breast lobules into the capillaries (described previously) and flows into the subareolar plexus, also known as the Sappey plexus.[26] The drainage continues to the axillary nodes approximately 75% of the time. Less commonly, the lymphatics drain medially to the internal mammary chain or deep to the retromammary lymphatics.

Imaging Technique

Mammography is the most common imaging modality used to evaluate the breast. **Table 1** outlines the appropriate tests for women of normal risk to develop breast cancer for both screening and diagnostic indications. For a woman over 40 years of age, a mammogram is the appropriate first-line test for both routine screening and for the diagnostic evaluation of a palpable mass.[27,28] **Fig. 4** shows a 59-year-old woman who had bilateral developing asymmetries detected on a screening

Table 1 Imaging protocols		
	Women Less Than 30–39 y of Age	**Women Greater Than or Equal to 40 y of Age**
Screening examination	None	Mammogram
Diagnostic examination	Ultrasound	Mammogram

Initial screening and diagnostic (for palpable lump) imaging tests for women of normal risk for developing breast cancer.

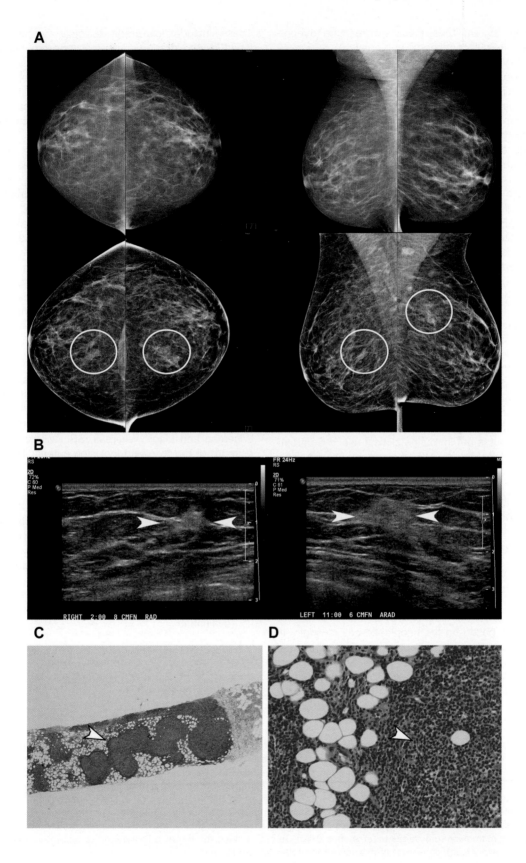

mammogram. These masses were found to represent follicular lymphoma at biopsy.

In younger women, less than 39 years of age, or those with a recent normal mammogram who have a palpable mass, ultrasound is the more appropriate initial imaging study.[28] **Fig. 5** shows bilateral ultrasound images of palpable masses (rapidly enlarging bilateral breasts) in a 25-year-old woman status post–stem cell transplant 1 year ago for recurrent B-acute lymphoblastic lymphoma (B-ALL). She was found to have recurrent B-ALL.

No distinct mammographic or ultrasonographic imaging features are known that would differentiate BL from a primary breast cancer.[29] The imaging features overlap with both invasive ductal and lobular carcinomas and sarcomatous masses and fibromatosis.[29] For this reason, an image-guided or physical examination–directed needle biopsy is necessary. The various modalities that can lead to an accurate diagnosis include fine-needle aspiration, core needle biopsy, and flow cytometry.[30,31]

After a diagnosis of BL, CT-PET scan is used for staging purposes. CT-PET has been shown superior to contrast-enhanced CT. **Fig. 5** shows a staging CT-PET in a 25-year-old patient with recurrent B-cell lymphoma. PET–MR imaging is currently being evaluated for its role in staging ENL but is not in routine clinical use.[32] Contrast-enhanced breast MR imaging is not routinely done in women with BL, in contrast to women with newly diagnosed breast cancer, in whom MR imaging is an appropriate next-line imaging study.[33]

IMAGING FINDINGS/PATHOLOGY

Lymphomas are categorized as Hodgkin lymphoma or non-Hodgkin lymphoma (NHL), with NHL more common in the breast (**Table 2**). NHL is further subdivided as either B cell or T cell, based on the neoplastic cell of origin. In general, B-cell lymphomas may be subdivided into low-grade and high-grade tumors. Generally, low-grade tumors tend to be comprised of small cells and have a more indolent course.

These include low-grade follicular lymphoma (see **Fig. 4**), extranodal marginal zone lymphoma (ENMZL) of mucosa-associated lymphoid tissue, small lymphocytic lymphoma, and lymphoplasmacytic lymphoma. Mantle cell lymphoma is an exception, in that typical cases have small to medium sized cells, but a more aggressive course.

High-grade tumors have medium to large cells with high mitotic activity and frequent tissue necrosis. The prototypical high-grade B-cell lymphoma is DLBCL (see **Fig. 1**). Several variants exist, depending on tumor site, phenotypic features, and patient immune status. Plasmablastic lymphoma and Burkitt lymphoma (see **Fig. 2**) are other examples of high-grade tumors.

T-cell lymphoma is rare in the breast (**Fig. 6**). A T-cell lymphoma of importance to breast imagers is anaplastic large cell lymphoma (ALCL). This disease occurs in the fibrous capsule of an implant and not typically from the breast parenchyma. It is seen in women with breast implants.

Diagnostic Criteria

Diagnostic considerations for PBL and SBL are similar and thus are discussed together.[3,15,34–36] PBL must meet the criteria initially described by Wiseman and Liao.[7] Whereas, SBL will break 1 or more of the following inclusion criteria. These criteria include.

- Closely associated mammary tissue and lymphomatous infiltrate
- Lack of synchronous disseminated lymphoma (the presence of ipsilateral axillary lymph node involvement is allowable under the category of PBL as long as this finding developed simultaneously[7])
- Lack of prior diagnosis of lymphoma
- An adequate specimen for pathologic evaluation

Using these criteria, PBL represents between 0.04% and 0.5% of primary breast malignancies,[14,37,38] 2.2% of ENLs,[37,39] and less than 1% of all NHLs.[19,38] Most patients with PBL

Fig. 4. (*A*) Screening-detected secondary involvement of the breast by follicular lymphoma. Current (*bottom* images) screening mammogram (*circles*) demonstrates bilateral developing asymmetries, a less common imaging appearance of BL, in the upper inner quadrants compared with a screening mammogram from 7 years prior (*top* mammogram). (*B*) Diagnostic work-up with mammography (not shown) and targeted bilateral ultrasound (*arrowheads*) confirmed masses in both breasts. The ultrasound shows a nontypical imaging appearance of lymphoma with bilateral oval, indistinct, hyperechoic masses with subtle posterior acoustic shadowing. (*C*) Hematoxylin-eosin stain at low power of the core biopsy specimen shows a distinct nodular proliferation infiltrating mammary adipose tissue (*arrowhead*). (*D*) On high power, the tumor cells are seen to be predominantly small (*arrowhead*), consistent with a low-grade follicular lymphoma.

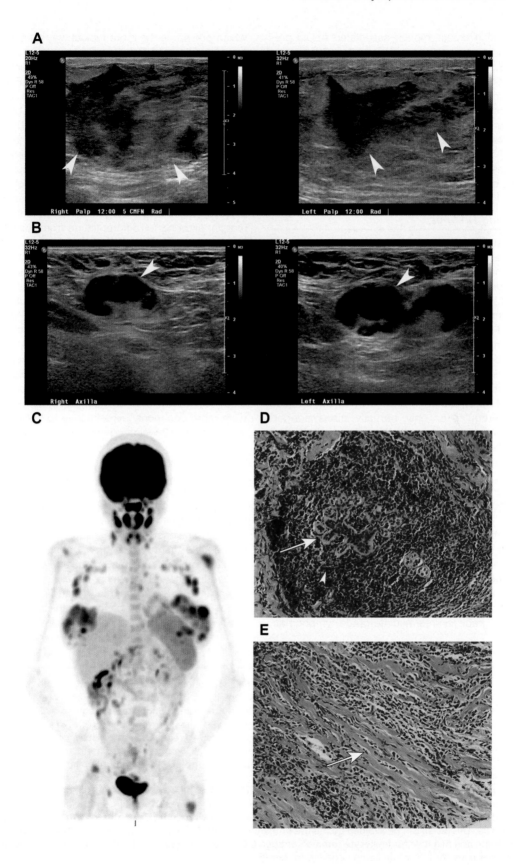

(excluding breast implant–associated ALCL) present with a palpable mass in the 5th or 6th decade of life.[2,9,16–18] The palpable finding is most often a solitary mass (see **Fig. 1**) but the disease can be multifocal or multicentric.[36] Findings, such as skin retraction, nipple involvement, and erythema, are rare.[40] **Fig. 7** demonstrates a neglected B-cell lymphoma with associated skin changes. A majority of SBLs are of B-cell type. Rare T-cell lymphomas, not associated with breast implants, have been reported.[41]

Imaging Findings

The imaging findings of BL are not specific and overlap with those of breast cancer.[36] The imaging findings also overlap between secondary BL and primary BL. The most common appearance of BL on mammography is a solitary, round, or oval mass with relatively circumscribed margins (see **Figs. 1** and **7**; **Figs. 8** and **9**).[42–45] It is uncommon for BL masses to have spiculated margins or associated microcalcifications.[17,43,46] In 12.5% of cases in the study of Sabate and colleagues,[36] the masses mimicked benign lesions (see **Fig. 9**), although a majority of the masses had irregular or only partially circumscribed margins. Other investigators have described diffuse increased opacity with or without skin thickening on mammography in 9% to 33% of cases.[17,36,42] In fewer than 10% of cases, BL presents as architectural distortion or an asymmetry (see **Fig. 4**). And in 3% to 13% of patients with BL, no abnormality is seen on mammography.[17,44,45]

A few studies have found a correlation between the imaging features on mammography with the histopathologic type of BL. High-grade lymphoma has been noted to more commonly present as diffuse breast enlargement (see **Fig. 5**) in contrast to low-grade or intermediate-grade lymphomas,

which present in the more typical way as a mass or asymmetry (see **Fig. 4**).[17,36,47]

On ultrasound, BL most commonly presents as a hypoechoic round or oval mass.[42,45] **Fig. 1** shows this typical imaging appearance in a woman who presented with a palpable right breast mass worked-up with mammography and ultrasound. Occasionally, on ultrasound, the masses can be so hypoechoic that they can be mistaken for cysts[42,44]; care must be taken to evaluate a finding to not mistake it for a benign or probably benign lesion. In approximately half of cases, the masses have mixed echogenicity or an indistinct margin, allowing for differentiation from a cyst or fibroadenoma.[45] **Fig. 4** shows a less common appearance of BL on ultrasound because this patient's masses were hyperechoic. Lyou and colleagues[43] reported a single case as hyperechoic on ultrasound. BL tends to be hypervascular on Doppler evaluation (see **Figs. 2** and **9**), which can also help exclude a cyst from the differential.[42]

There are few reports of BL on breast MR imaging; the rarity of reports is likely due to the fact that breast MR imaging is not the study of choice for staging. In 23 lesions in 8 patients, reported in a study by Sorov and colleagues,[45] the lesions were more commonly hyperintense to breast parenchyma on T2-weighted images and isointense on T1-weighted images. The masses had homogeneous internal enhancement patterns with rapid initial and mixed delayed kinetics (see **Fig. 2**). These features are not unique to BL.

Most lesions are also oval or round with circumscribed margins on CT (see **Fig. 8**). Again, these imaging findings are nonspecific and do not differentiate them from a breast cancer, cyst, or fibroadenoma. If contrast is given, lymphoma, fibroadenoma, and breast cancer all are expected to enhance to some degree. When imaged with PET, BL and breast cancer both are known to have increased fluorodeoxyglucose F 18

Fig. 5. Secondary involvement of the breasts by recurrent B-cell lymphoma. A 25-year-old woman with history of acute lymphoblastic lymphoma status post–stem cell transplant 1 year prior presented with rapid onset bilateral breast fullness with pain under both arms. (*A*) Bilateral breast ultrasound demonstrates irregular, indistinct, heterogeneous masses throughout all quadrants of the bilateral breasts (images from the 12 o'clock region of both breasts [*arrowheads*]). (*B*) Bilateral axillary ultrasounds reveal bilateral adenopathy (*arrowheads*). She underwent right breast and axillary biopsy confirming recurrent extranodal B-cell lymphoma. After her diagnosis, a staging CT-PET scan was performed, showing widespread abnormal ^{18}F-FDG uptake (*C*) in multiple bilateral axillary and levels III and IV, periportal, and right superficial inguinal lymph nodes and in both breasts, the spleen, the bilateral humeral heads, right acetabular roof, left femoral neck, and the bilateral distal femurs and proximal tibias. (*D*) Hematoxylin-eosin at medium power shows tumor cells (*arrowhead*) surrounding epithelial structures (*arrow*). (*E*) Higher power highlights linear arrays of tumor cells (*arrow*) that may be confused with invasive lobular carcinoma. This pitfall can be avoided by the use of immunohistochemical stains. Carcinoma cells will be positive for keratin and negative for leukocyte common antigen (LCA), also referred to as CD45. Lymphoma cells demonstrate positivity for LCA while being negative for keratin.

Table 2
Pathology summary of lymphoma subtypes that can affect the breast

Morphology	Important Considerations
B-cell lymphomas	
B-ALL	
Diffuse proliferation of small to large cells with fine, immature chromatin and elevated mitotic activity	Immunohistochemistry or flow cytometry is needed to differentiate B-cell from T-cell process
Burkitt lymphoma	
Diffuse infiltrate of medium-sized cells with multiple small to medium nucleoli, clumped and dispersed chromatin, and lipid containing vacuoles in the cytoplasm Markedly elevated mitotic activity	Bilateral breast disease can be seen during pregnancy/lactation or puberty
Chronic lymphocytic leukemia/small lymphocytic lymphoma	
Comprised of small, round lymphocytes, usually with clumped chromatin and indistinct nucleoli Tends to grow in diffuse sheets with vague nodularity	Often have proliferation centers, which consist of larger cells, which may lead to confusion with a high-grade process
DLBCL	
Diffuse proliferation of large atypical lymphocytes, with large, variably vesicular nuclei and 1 or multiple prominent nucleoli	Most common type of PBL
ENMZL of mucosa-associated lymphoid tissue	
Small atypical lymphocytes, often with clear cytoplasm, frequently accompanied by a variable number of plasma cells Low mitotic activity	These tumors can be inconspicuous and can be mistaken for a benign inflammatory process
Follicular lymphoma	
Nodular proliferation is characteristic Low-grade tumors are comprised predominantly of small lymphocytes with irregular nuclear contours and indistinct nucleoli (centrocytes). Higher-grade tumors have an increased population of larger cells with multiple distinct nucleoli (centroblasts).	Careful assessment is necessary to rule out an associated DLBCL component
Lymphoplasmacytic lymphoma	
Proliferation of small lymphocytes, plasmacytoid lymphocytes, and plasma cells	Can be associated with Waldenström macroglobulinemia
Mantle cell lymphoma	
Small cells with irregular nuclear contours and indistinct nucleoli Variable mitotic activity	The blastoid variant is a more aggressive form where tumor cells resemble lymphoblasts and have increased mitotic activity
Plasmablastic lymphoma	
Diffuse proliferation of large atypical cells with prominent nucleoli and increased mitotic activity Variable plasmacytoid morphology (can have some resemblance to plasma cells)	Typically seen in immunocompromised patients, highly associated with HIV and Epstein-Barr virus, and most frequently seen in the oral cavity
B-cell markers: CD20, CD19, CD79a, Pax5	
T-cell lymphomas	
ALCL	
Diffuse proliferation of large atypical cells with cohesive growth that can resemble carcinoma cells	Associated with breast implants Immunohistochemistry can be helpful to differentiate from carcinoma, which is keratin positive

(continued on next page)

Table 2
(continued)

Morphology	Important Considerations
T lymphoblastic leukemia/lymphoma	
Diffuse proliferation of small to large cells with fine, immature chromatin and elevated mitotic activity	Immunohistochemistry or flow cytometry is needed to differentiate B-cell from T-cell process
T-cell markers: CD3, CD2, CD5, CD7, CD4, CD8, CD1a	
Others	
Hodgkin lymphoma	
Proliferation consists predominantly of background non-neoplastic cells, including small lymphocytes, plasma cells, eosinophils, neutrophils, and histiocytes. Tumor cells are large, often with 2 nuclei, and have prominent nucleoli (Reed-Sternberg cells)	Malignant cells are a minority of the tumor mass; thus, techniques, such as flow cytometry, which rely on defining relatively larger populations of cells, are not diagnostic
Plasmacytoma	
Diffuse sheets of plasma cells with variable cellular atypia and mitotic activity	Must distinguish from a low-grade lymphoma with plasmacytoid morphology, in particularl ENMZL Small percentage can progress to plasma cell myeloma

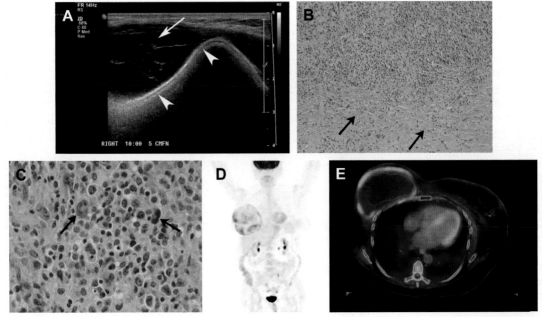

Fig. 6. ALCL. (*A*) Ultrasound in a patient status post–remote right mastectomy with silicone implant reconstruction 20 years prior, implant exchange to saline 6 years prior, who presented with 1-week right breast swelling and discomfort, shows a large complex fluid collection (*arrow*) around the implant (*arrowheads*). Patient denied any recent right breast procedures and was not on anticoagulation. (*B*) Hematoxylin-eosin stain of biopsy of the fibrous capsule at low power demonstrates atypical lymphocytes associated with fibrous capsule (*arrows*). Note in this image the lack of mammary epithelial or adipose tissue. (*C*) Hematoxylin-eosin stain at high power better shows the large atypical lymphocytes, including hallmark cells (*arrows*), which often have a horseshoe appearance. (*D*, MIP, and *E*, CT-PET) The patient later underwent a demonstrating abnormal ^{18}F-FDG uptake seen in the fibrous capsule surrounding the fluid and implant without other evidence of disease.

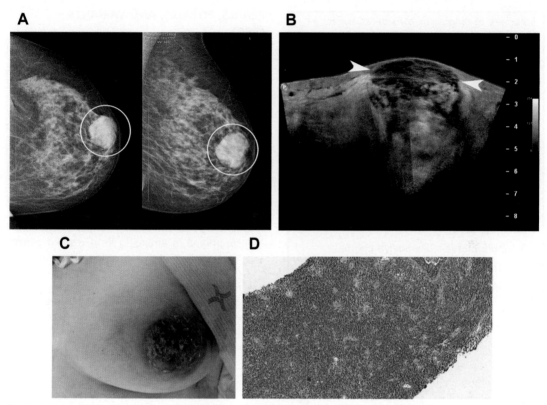

Fig. 7. Advanced B-cell lymphoma presenting as a mass with overlying skin ulceration. (*A*) Mammogram shows a round, indistinct, equal-density mass (*circles*). (*B*) Ultrasound demonstrates an oval, indistinct, heterogeneous mass extending to the skin surface (*arrowheads*). (*C*) An image of the patient shows the ulcerated skin overlying the subareolar mass. (*D*) Hematoxylin-eosin stain at low power shows the typical appearance of a lower-grade tumor with sheet of small cells.

(^{18}F-FDG) uptake compared with background parenchymal tissue. Both local and diffuse uptake has been described in cases of BL.[48,49] PET or CT-PET can help evaluate for the presence or absence of disease outside the breast and is useful in staging BL. **Fig. 8** shows the expected increased ^{18}F-FDG uptake in the oval, circumscribed right breast mass that is typically seen in BL. **Figs. 5** and **6** demonstrate the utility of PET-CT for staging lymphoma and documenting the presence or absence of disease outside the breast.

ALCL of the breast is rare but deserves discussion because the presentation differs from the more typical B-cell lymphoma. Only 6% of BLs have morphologic and immunohistochemical features consistent with ALCL.[50] According to a Food and Drug Administration 2011 report, there is a possible association between breast implants and ALCL, although the incidence is low. Approximately 1 in 500, 000 women with breast implants develop implant-associated ALCL.[51,52] And both saline and silicone implants have been implicated.[41] Most patients present with an effusion around the implant and contained

within a fibrous capsule (see **Fig. 6**).[51] A distinct mass associated with effusion can also be seen but is less common. ALCL associated with breast implants is usually, but not exclusively, unilateral.[53]

Differential diagnosis
PBL
SBL
Breast cancer
Invasive ductal carcinoma, not otherwise specified
Medullary carcinoma
Mucinous carcinoma
Fibroadenoma
Cyst
Sarcomatous neoplasm
Fibromatosis

Summary of diagnostic considerations for breast lymphomas
B-cell lymphomas
DLBCL
Follicular lymphoma
ENMZL
Mantle cell lymphoma
Lymphoplasmacytic lymphoma
Plasmablastic lymphoma
B lymphoblastic leukemia/lymphoma
Small lymphocytic lymphoma
T-cell lymphomas
T lymphoblastic leukemia/lymphoma
Cutaneous T-cell lymphoma
Breast implant–associated lymphoma
ALCL

PEARLS, PITFALLS, AND VARIANTS
Pearls

- The breast is an uncommon location for ENL. Overall leukemia and lymphoma, however, are the most common sources of extramammary cancer involving the breast.
- Secondary involvement of the breast by known lymphoma is more common than PBL. When primary, B-cell lymphoma, specifically DLBCL, is most common.
- Women with PBL typically present with a solitary palpable breast mass visible on diagnostic mammogram and/or ultrasound indistinguishable from a breast cancer.
- Although still uncommon, implant-associated lymphoma is emerging as a distinct clinical entity and is seen in women with either silicone or saline implants.
- Fine-needle aspiration, core needle biopsy, and flow cytometry are valuable diagnostic approaches to secure an accurate diagnosis and avoid mistreatment.

A

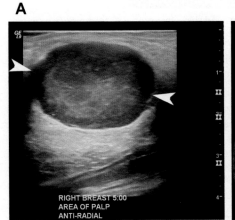

B

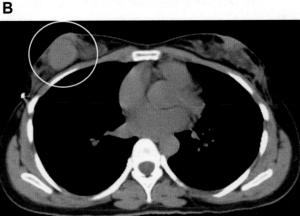

C

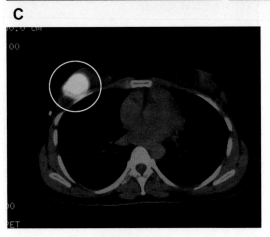

Fig. 8. B-cell lymphoma presenting as a palpable right breast mass. (*A*) The mass demonstrates the typical ultrasound appearance as an oval, circumscribed, homogeneously hypoechoic solid mass (*arrowheads*). (*B*) On nonenhanced axial chest CT and (*C*) correlative slice on PET-CT, the mass also has an oval shape with circumscribed margins (*circles*). (*C*) The mass has diffuse homogeneous increased 18F-FDG uptake as is commonly seen in lymphoma on PET (*circle*).

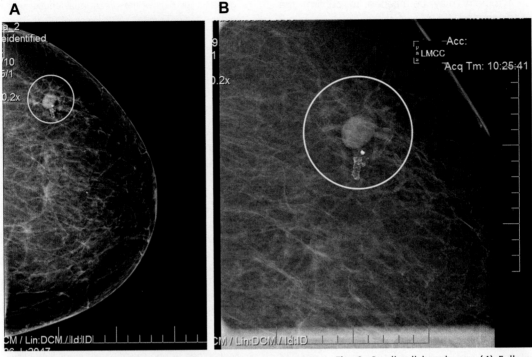

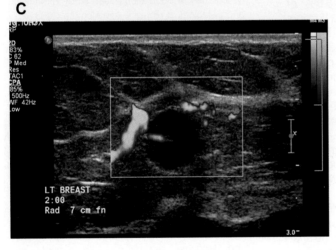

Fig. 9. Small cell lymphoma. (*A*) Full craniocaudal view and (*B*) spot magnification craniocaudal view show the typical appearance of BL with an oval, circumscribed equal-density mass on mammography (*circles*). (*C*) On ultrasound, the mass is markedly hypoechoic with associated increased vascularity on Doppler imaging. These imaging findings are nonspecific for BL. Note how the mass has a relatively benign appearance on the imaging.

Pitfalls

- Clinical presentation and imaging appearance of BL mimic breast carcinoma.
- Imaging appearance of BL occasionally overlaps with benign cysts or fibroadenomas, leading to incorrect assessment as a benign or probably benign finding.
- Misinterpretation of atypical hematopoietic cells as carcinoma cells may lead to an erroneous diagnosis and incorrect treatment. In particular, individual infiltrating lymphoma cells may be misinterpreted as invasive lobular carcinoma, and morphologic similarities with

medullary carcinoma may also pose a problem.

- Rarely, lymphomatous involvement of the breast may present with breast skin thickening, induration, and edema, suggestive of peau d'orange changes. Histologic evaluation and ancillary immunohistochemistry testing, if necessary, rule out an inflammatory carcinoma.
- Pathologic overlap with more benign histologies can create difficulties. Ancillary techniques, such as immunohistochemistry, fluorescence in situ hybridization, and flow

cytometry may be needed to confirm the diagnoses.

WHAT THE REFERRING PHYSICIAN NEEDS TO KNOW

- Patients with a new palpable breast mass should be referred for breast imaging.
- If a patient has a history of lymphoma, recurrence in the setting of a new breast mass on screening mammography or physical examination needs to be considered.
- A biopsy should be performed for any mass deemed probably benign if it increases in size on physical examination or on follow-up imaging.
- Treatment of BL is different than for breast carcinoma, and referral to hematology/oncology is an appropriate next step after diagnosis.

SUMMARY

Lymphoma is the most common extramammary breast cancer and occurs most often in the 5th to 6th decades. It is usually secondary to systemic lymphoma and represents less than 0.5% of breast malignancy. Primary lymphoma occurs less commonly but presents similarly. The most common type for both primary and secondary lymphoma is B cell, although any cell type is possible.

BL most often presents as a nonspecific breast mass. In cases of PBL, invasive ductal carcinoma is usually the prebiopsy diagnosis. When lymphoma is already present, it may be included in the differential.

The diagnosis is made by biopsy and treatment is chemotherapy and radiation, not surgical excision. The outcome is less favorable, however, than that for epithelial breast cancer.

Lymphoma in the breast should not be forgotten as the cause of breast disease, even though it is rare. Knowledge of its pathology and imaging findings are necessary for its diagnosis and treatment.

REFERENCES

1. Zucca E, Roggero E, Bertoni F, et al. Primary extranodal non-hodgkin's lymphomas. part 2: Head and neck, central nervous system and other less common sites. Ann Oncol 1999;10:1023–33.
2. Bobrow LG, Richards MA, Happerfield LC, et al. Breast lymphomas: A clinicopathologic review. Hum Pathol 1993;24(3):274–8.
3. Duncan VE, Reddy VV, Jhala NC, et al. Non-hodgkin's lymphoma of the breast: A review of 18 primary and secondary cases. Ann Diagn Pathol 2006;10(3):144–8.
4. Tavassoli FA, Devilee P, editors. World health organization classification of tumours. Pathology &

genetics tumours of the breast and female genital organs. Lyon (France): IARC Press; 2003.
5. Hugh JC, Jackson FI, Hanson J, et al. Primary breast lymphoma. an immunohistologic study of 20 new cases. Cancer 1990;66(12):2602–11.
6. Adair FE, Hermann JB. Primary lymphosarcoma of the breast. Surgery 1944;16:836–53.
7. Wiseman C, Liao KT. Primary lymphoma of the breast. Cancer 1972;29(6):1705–12.
8. Mpallas G, Simatos G, Tasidou A, et al. Primary breast lymphoma in a male patient. Breast 2004; 13(5):436–8.
9. Wong WW, Schild SE, Halyard MY, et al. Primary non-hodgkin lymphoma of the breast: The mayo clinic experience. J Surg Oncol 2002;80(1):19–25 [discussion: 26].
10. Brustein S, Filippa DA, Kimmel M, et al. Malignant lymphoma of the breast. A study of 53 patients. Ann Surg 1987;205(2):144–50.
11. Ha CS, Dubey P, Goyal LK, et al. Localized primary non-hodgkin lymphoma of the breast. Am J Clin Oncol 1998;21(4):376–80.
12. Kuper-Hommel MJ, Snijder S, Janssen-Heijnen ML, et al. Treatment and survival of 38 female breast lymphomas: A population-based study with clinical and pathological reviews. Ann Hematol 2003;82(7): 397–404.
13. Jennings WC, Baker RS, Murray SS, et al. Primary breast lymphoma: The role of mastectomy and the importance of lymph node status. Ann Surg 2007; 245(5):784–9.
14. Earnest RE, Downey DM, Fox JP, et al. Recurrence of primary breast lymphoma in contralateral breast: Case report and review of the literature. J Surg Educ 2008;65(5):364–6.
15. Domchek SM, Hecht JL, Fleming MD, et al. Lymphomas of the breast: Primary and secondary involvement. Cancer 2002;94(1):6–13.
16. Jeon HJ, Akagi T, Hoshida Y, et al. Primary non-hodgkin malignant lymphoma of the breast. an immunohistochemical study of seven patients and literature review of 152 patients with breast lymphoma in Japan. Cancer 1992;70(10): 2451–9.
17. Liberman L, Giess CS, Dershaw DD, et al. Non-hodgkin lymphoma of the breast: Imaging characteristics and correlation with histopathologic findings. Radiology 1994;192:157–60.
18. Feder JM, Shaw de Paredes E, Hogge JP, et al. Unusual breast lesions: radiologic-pathologic correlation. Radiographics 1999;19:S11–26.
19. Validire P, Capovilla M, Asselain B, et al. Primary breast non-hodgkin's lymphoma: A large single center study of initial characteristics, natural history, and prognostic factors. Am J Hematol 2009;84(3):133–9.
20. National Cancer Institute. SEER cancer statistics factsheets: breast cancer. Bethesda (MD). Available

at: http://seer.cancer.gov/statfacts/html/breast.html. Accessed August 20, 2015.

21. Early Breast Cancer Trialists' Collaborative Group (EBCTCG). Effect of radiotherapy after breast-conserving surgery on 10-year recurrence and 15-year breast cancer death: Meta-analysis of individual patient data for 10,801 women in 17 randomised trials. Lancet 2011;378(9804):1707–16.

22. Sadler TW. Langman's medical embryology. 5th edition. Baltimore (MD): Williams & Wilkins; 1985.

23. Wellings SR. A hypothesis of the origin of human breast cancer from the terminal ductal lobular unit. Pathol Res Pract 1980;166(5):515–35.

24. Schmid-Schonbein GW. Microlymphatics and lymph flow. Physiol Rev 1990;70:987–1028.

25. Tanis PJ, Nieweg OE, Valdés Olmos RA, et al. Anatomy and physiology of lymphatic drainage of the breast from the perspective of sentinel node biopsy1. J Am Coll Surg 2001;192(3):399–409.

26. Turner-Warwick RT. The lymphatics of the breast. Br J Surg 1959;46:574–82.

27. American College of Radiology. American college of radiology appropriateness criteria, breast cancer screening. 2012. Available at: https://acsearch.acr.org/docs/70910/Narrative/. Accessed August 20, 2015.

28. American College of Radiology. American college of radiology appropriateness criteria, palpable breast masses. 2012. Available at: https://acsearch.acr.org/docs/69495/Narrative/. Accessed August 20, 2015.

29. Schillaci O, Travascio L, Lacanfora A, et al. Rare lymphoid malignancies of the breast: Report of two cases illustrating potential diagnostic techniques. J Radiol Case Rep 2012;6(12):43–50.

30. Martinelli G, Ryan G, Seymour JF, et al. Primary follicular and marginal-zone lymphoma of the breast: Clinical features, prognostic factors and outcome: a study by the international extranodal lymphoma study group. Ann Oncol 2009;20(12):1993–9.

31. Sharma S, Dorwal P, Sachdev R, et al. Primary follicular lymphoma of the breast: A rare clinical entity diagnosed using tissue flow cytometry. Indian J Hematol Blood Transfus 2015;31(2):300–1.

32. Heacock L, Weissbrot J, Raad R, et al. PET/MRI for the evaluation of patients with lymphoma: Initial observation. AJR Am J Roentgenol 2015;204(4):842–8.

33. Houssami N, Ciatto S, Macaskill P, et al. Accuracy and surgical impact of magnetic resonance imaging in breast cancer staging: Systematic review and meta-analysis in detection of multifocal and multicentric cancer. J Clin Oncol 2008;26(19):3248–58.

34. Samoon Z, Idrees R, Masood N, et al. Plasmablastic lymphoma of the oral cavity with breast recurrence: A case report. BMC Res Notes 2015;8:180.

35. Talwalkar SS, Miranda RN, Valbuena JR, et al. Lymphomas involving the breast: A study of 106 cases comparing localized and disseminated neoplasms. Am J Surg Pathol 2008;32(9):1299–309.

36. Sabate JM, Gomez A, Torrubia S, et al. Lymphoma of the breast: Clinical and radiologic features with pathologic correlation in 28 patients. Breast J 2002;8(5):294–304.

37. Mouna B, Saber B, Tijani el H, et al. Primary malignant non-hodgkin's lymphoma of the breast: A study of seven cases and literature review. World J Surg Oncol 2012;10:151.

38. Romero-Guadarrama MB, Hernandez-Gonzalez MM, Duran-Padilla MA, et al. Primary lymphomas of the breast: A report on 5 cases studied in a period of 5 years at the hospital general de mexico. Ann Diagn Pathol 2009;13(2):78–81.

39. Roden AC, Macon WR, Keeney GL, et al. Seroma-associated primary anaplastic large-cell lymphoma adjacent to breast implants: An indolent T-cell lymphoproliferative disorder. Mod Pathol 2008;21(4):455–63.

40. Ho CW, Mantoo S, Lim CH, et al. Synchronous invasive ductal carcinoma and intravascular large B-cell lymphoma of the breast: A case report and review of the literature. World J Surg Oncol 2014;12:88.

41. Lazzeri D, Agostini T, Bocci G, et al. ALK-1-negative anaplastic large cell lymphoma associated with breast implants: A new clinical entity. Clin Breast Cancer 2011;11(5):283–96.

42. Yang WT, Lane DL, Le-Petross HT, et al. Breast lymphoma: Imaging findings of 32 tumors in 27 patients. Radiology 2007;245(3):692–702.

43. Lyou CY, Yang SK, Choe DH, et al. Mammographic and sonographic findings of primary breast lymphoma. Clin Imaging 2007;31(4):234–8.

44. Jackson FI, Lalani ZH. Breast lymphoma: Radiologic imaging and clinical appearances. Can Assoc Radiol J 1991;42(1):48–54.

45. Surov A, Holzhausen H, Wienke A, et al. Primary and secondary breast lymphoma: Prevalence, clinical signs and radiological features. Br J Radiol 2012;85(1014):e195–205.

46. Paulus DD. Lymphoma of the breast. Radiol Clin North Am 1990;28(4):833–40.

47. Meyer JE, Kopans DB, Long JC. Mammographic appearance of malignant lymphoma of the breast. Radiology 1980;135(3):623–6.

48. Nihashi T, Hayasaka K, Itou T, et al. Findings of fluorine-18-FDG PET in extranodal origin lymphoma–in three cases of diffuse large B cell typelymphoma. Ann Nucl Med 2006;20(10):689–93.

49. Kumar R, Xiu Y, Dhurairaj T, et al. F-18 FDG positron emission tomography in non-hodgkin lymphoma of the breast. Clin Nucl Med 2005;30(4):246–8.

50. Popplewell L, Thomas SH, Huang Q, et al. Primary anaplastic large-cell lymphoma associated with breast implants. Leuk Lymphoma 2011;52(8):1481–7.

51. Miranda RN, Aladily TN, Prince HM, et al. Breast implant-associated anaplastic large-cell lymphoma: Long-term follow-up of 60 patients. J Clin Oncol 2014;32(2):114–20.

52. Lee YS, Filie A, Arthur D, et al. Breast-implant-associated anaplastic large cell lymphoma in a patient with li-fraumeni syndrome. Histopathology 2015; 67(6):925–7.

53. Bautista-Quach MA, Nademanee A, Weisenburger DD, et al. Implant-associated primary anaplastic large-cell lymphoma with simultaneous involvement of bilateral breast capsules. Clin Breast Cancer 2013;13(6):492–5.

Pediatric Extranodal Lymphoma

Ellen M. Chung, MD[a,b,*], Michael Pavio, BS[c]

KEYWORDS

- Lymphoma • Children • Non-Hodgkin lymphoma • Burkitt lymphoma • Lymphoblastic lymphoma
- Diffuse large B-cell lymphoma • Anaplastic large cell lymphoma

KEY POINTS

- Compared with non-Hodgkin lymphoma (NHL) in adults, the histologic spectrum of pediatric disease is quite narrow and consists of aggressive forms causing widespread disease.
- Burkitt lymphoma is the most common type of pediatric NHL and the most common site of involvement is the ileocecal region, often presenting acutely with intussusception.
- Lymphoblastic lymphoma, as well as other types of NHL, can manifest with rapidly enlarging mediastinal masses causing compression of the airway and superior vena cava.
- Staging and assessment of treatment response are usually performed with fluorodeoxyglucose (FDG)-PET/computed tomography, although alternative techniques with no or lower radiation dose are being evaluated.

Lymphoma is the third most common pediatric neoplasm after leukemia and central nervous system (CNS) tumors, accounting for 10% to 15% of cancers in children. In the United States seven hundred new cases are diagnosed annually, nearly half of which are non-Hodgkin lymphomas (NHLs).[1] NHL is more often extranodal in children than is Hodgkin lymphoma or NHL in adults. NHL shows a predilection for male and white patients and is more common than Hodgkin disease in children younger than 10 years of age.[1]

Pediatric NHL differs from adult disease. NHL that affects children is far less varied in histology and more likely to derive from primitive precursor cells.[2] Disease is typically widespread at presentation in children, and indolent types of lymphoma seen in adults do not occur in pediatric patients. Only 4 types of NHL commonly occur in children: Burkitt lymphoma, lymphoblastic lymphoma, diffuse large B-cell lymphoma (DLBCL), and anaplastic large cell lymphoma (ALCL).

BURKITT LYMPHOMA

Burkitt lymphoma is an aggressive mature B-cell lymphoma and the most common subtype of NHL in children, accounting for 40% of cases in the United States.[3] Burkitt lymphoma primarily involves extranodal sites and, as one of the fastest growing malignancies, generally presents with widespread disease.[4,5] There is a strong male predilection with a male-to-female ratio of 4 to 1. The

The opinions and assertions contained herein are the private views of the authors and are not to be construed as official or as representing the views of the Departments of the Army or Defense.

Disclosure Statement: The authors have nothing to disclose.

[a] Department of Radiology and Radiological Sciences, F. Edward Hébert School of Medicine, Uniformed Services University of the Health Sciences, 4301 Jones Bridge Road, Bethesda, MD 20814, USA; [b] Pediatric Radiology Section, American Institute for Radiologic Pathology, Silver Spring, MD 20190, USA; [c] F. Edward Hébert School of Medicine, Uniformed Services University of the Health Sciences, 4301 Jones Bridge Road, Bethesda, MD 20814, USA

* Corresponding author. Department of Radiology and Radiological Sciences, Uniformed Services University of the Health Sciences, 4301 Jones Bridge Road, Bethesda, MD 20814.

E-mail address: ellen.chung@usuhs.edu

Radiol Clin N Am 54 (2016) 727–746
http://dx.doi.org/10.1016/j.rcl.2016.03.004
0033-8389/16/$ – see front matter Published by Elsevier Inc.

age range is 0 to 20 years with a median age of 8 years. Children between the ages of 5 to 9 comprise more than one-third of cases.[3]

The tumor is named for the surgeon, Denis Parsons Burkitt, who identified a group of children with rapidly enlarging jaw masses while working in Uganda.[6] The World Health Organization now recognizes 3 clinical variants: endemic, sporadic, and immunodeficiency-related Burkitt lymphoma.[7]

The endemic type afflicts children in equatorial Africa and Papua New Guinea where it is the most common childhood malignancy. The peak age of incidence is 4 to 7 years.[7] Endemic Burkitt lymphoma is an Epstein-Barr virus (EBV)-mediated tumor; nearly all tumors (95%) are latently infected.[8] Additionally, the geographic distribution of the endemic form overlaps with that of malaria, although the relationship between malaria, EBV, and Burkitt lymphoma has not yet been fully elucidated. The disease usually involves the jaw and facial bones of young children with characteristic involvement of the developing molar teeth. Disease of the gastrointestinal (GI) tract, kidneys, bone, gonads, and breasts is also common. CNS and peripheral lymph node disease is less frequent.

The sporadic variant, previously known as American Burkitt lymphoma, occurs worldwide and also affects young adults. In the United States 500 cases are diagnosed annually.[9] There is a male predilection with a male-to-female ratio of 2–3 to 1 in adults, likely higher in children.[7] Associated EBV infection is found in 25% to 30% of cases.[5,8] Jaw tumors are rare in this form. The GI tract is most frequently involved and 30% to 40% of patients present with acute abdominal complaints mimicking acute appendicitis.[4,10,11]

The immunodeficiency-associated form occurs primarily in patients with human immunodeficiency virus (HIV) but also in patients with congenital immunodeficiency (eg, Wiskott-Aldrich syndrome, ataxia telangiectasia) and in allograft recipients. This is the most common subtype of lymphoma in children with HIV accounting for 40% of cases.[2] There is also an association with EBV infection, though less than in the endemic form, involving 25% to 40% of cases.[5,8] This association is higher for HIV-infected patients and solid organ transplant recipients.[12]

Pathology Findings

Macroscopically, a fleshy pink to tan mass frequently involving the bowel wall and encasing mesenteric vessels is seen (**Fig. 1**). Due to the short doubling time, central tumor necrosis is common.[4,11] At histology, the tumor consists of medium-sized, monomorphic cells with round or oval nuclei, coarse chromatin, several nucleoli, and a moderate amount of densely basophilic cytoplasm. High mitotic index is typical, along with many apoptotic cells, the nuclear remnants of which are ingested by macrophages. These pale tingible body macrophages are interspersed among the deeply basophilic tumor cells, creating the characteristic starry-sky pattern seen on light microscopy (**Fig. 2**).[7,13]

The tumor cells are of B-cell lineage and express mature B-cell markers: CD20, CD19, CD2, and CD79a. The morphologic and immunophenotypic features may be indistinguishable from those of DLBCL; however, genetic analysis reveals the characteristic t(8;14)(q24;q32) translocation that leads to deregulation of the c-MYC proto-oncogene.[5,9,14] The c-MYC coding sequence is partnered to strong immunoglobulin-promoter and enhancer elements, which drive its expression.[12]

Imaging Features

Extranodal sites are predominantly involved, typically with bulky disease. The most common site of involvement in sporadic and immunodeficiency-associated Burkitt lymphoma is the GI tract with abdominal and pelvic masses evident in 31% to 64% of cases.[4] The most frequently affected sites are distal ileum, cecum, and appendix, a predilection that is presumably due to the concentration of lymphoid tissue in these regions in the form of Peyer patches (see **Fig. 1**). The tumor spreads circumferentially from the submucosa and deep mucosal layers, manifesting as diffuse bowel wall thickening and/or as mural masses on imaging (**Fig. 3**). The mural masses may serve as pathology lead points for intussusception and Burkitt lymphoma is the most common cause of intussusception in children older than 4 years of age.[15] The bowel lumen may be either narrowed due to mass effect or dilated due to tumor invasion of the autonomic plexus and muscularis propria. The latter process disrupts peristalsis and leads to bowel wall dilation and an aneurysmal appearance that is characteristic of Burkitt lymphoma (see **Fig. 3**).[4,14,16] Enlarged abdominal lymph nodes may be seen.[2,17] Complications of tumor mass effect may be evident on imaging, including bowel, biliary, or ureteral obstruction. Malignant ascites is seen in up to one-quarter of cases.[4,11,15,18]

On ultrasound, tumor invasion of the bowel wall produces hypoechoic bowel wall thickening with loss of the normally stratified appearance. A focal hypoechoic, complex mass may be seen.[17] In

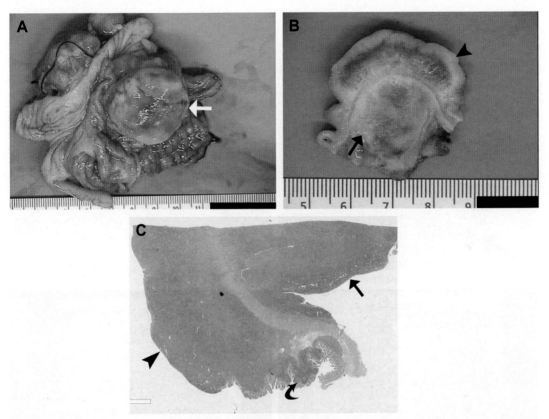

Fig. 1. Burkitt lymphoma in a 5-year-old boy. (*A*) Gross specimen shows a pink, fleshy mass (*arrow*) at the ileocecal valve. (*B*) Sectioned specimen reveals the tumor (*arrow*) infiltrates the bowel wall under the thickened mucosa (*arrowhead*). (*C*) Photomicrograph (H&E stain, low power) shows a diffuse lymphoid proliferation (*arrow*) infiltrating the bowel wall under the mucosa (*arrowhead*). Adjacent normal lymphoid tissue with germinal centers (Peyer patches) is seen (*curved arrow*).

cases of intussusception, the target or doughnut appearance of alternating concentric hyperechoic and hypoechoic lines representing bowel wall within bowel wall with central echogenic mesenteric fat is seen on compression ultrasound (see **Fig. 2**).

At computed tomography (CT), involved bowel is thickened with minimal enhancement. A focal mass with central hypoattenuating necrosis is a common appearance. A bulky mass representing disease extension into the mesentery is characteristic. Encasement of the mesenteric vessels is a common and distinctive finding.[4,14,15,19] A mesenteric mass surrounding the enhancing vessels produces an appearance known as the sandwich sign.[4,15,20] Calcifications are uncommon before treatment.[15] Peritoneal seeding is infrequent and appears as nodules along the liver capsule and peritoneal reflections and, rarely, as omental caking (**Fig. 4**).[15,21] At MR imaging, the masses are of homogenous, low signal intensity on T1-and heterogeneous, intermediate signal intensity on T2-weighted images (see **Fig. 3**). Mild enhancement following intravenous gadolinium chelate is seen.

Lymphomatous involvement of the solid abdominal organs may also occur. Hepatic involvement is seen in about 17% of cases (**Figs. 5 and 6**)[4] and disease of the liver usually occurs in conjunction with spleen involvement. Renal involvement is almost always related to disseminated disease and manifests as focal or multiple masses with preservation of the reniform shape (**Fig. 7**). Ovaries may also be affected (**Fig. 8**). In general, the involved organs may be enlarged with or without focal lesions. Focal masses appear hypoechoic to the adjacent parenchyma on ultrasound and hypoattenuating on contrast-enhanced CT.

Additional sites of involvement include the breasts, particularly during periods of hormonal stimulation such as puberty and pregnancy (**Fig. 9**). Disease is typically bulky and bilateral. Involvement of the mediastinum and pulmonary

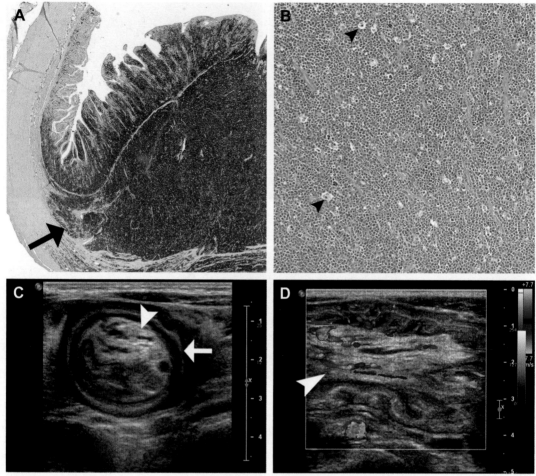

Fig. 2. Burkitt lymphoma causing ileocecal intussusception in a 4-year-old boy. (*A*) Photomicrograph (Ki-67 immunostain, original magnification 20×) demonstrates a mass infiltrating the bowel wall and mucosa with intense diffuse positive staining for Ki-67 indicating a high proliferative index (*arrow*). (*B*) Photomicrograph (H&E stain, intermediate power) shows a few large, pale tingible body macrophages (*arrowheads*) interspersed among diffuse small-size to intermediate-size basophilic cells, creating the starry-sky pattern. (*C*) Transverse ultrasound image in the right lower quadrant demonstrates concentric rings of alternating hyperechogenicity and hypoechogenicity (*arrow*) surrounding echogenic mesenteric fat (*arrowhead*), causing the doughnut sign. (*D*) Longitudinal ultrasound image with color Doppler reveals layered appearance with central echogenic mesenteric fat (*arrowhead*), the pseudokidney sign, and flow within vessels.

parenchyma is rare in Burkitt lymphoma. CNS involvement indicates stage IV disease and may occur in all variants.[7,22] Lesions may be solitary or diffuse with a predilection for the gray-white matter interface, basal ganglia, and periventricular white matter tracts. Enhancement is typically ring-like.[2]

LYMPHOBLASTIC LYMPHOMA

Almost all lymphoblastic lymphomas in children are derived from precursor T-cells. The disease is uncommon in adults but accounts for 30% of pediatric NHLs. Male patients are more commonly

affected.[1,7] By convention, if there is extensive involvement of the bone marrow (greater than 25%) or peripheral blood with blasts, then the disease is termed lymphoblastic leukemia. Other types of pediatric lymphoma less commonly present with a leukemic phase.

Clinical Considerations

Mediastinal mass is a common feature and rapid growth may cause compression of the trachea and bronchi and/or the superior vena cava. Such a presentation constitutes an oncologic emergency and a management dilemma. The clinical

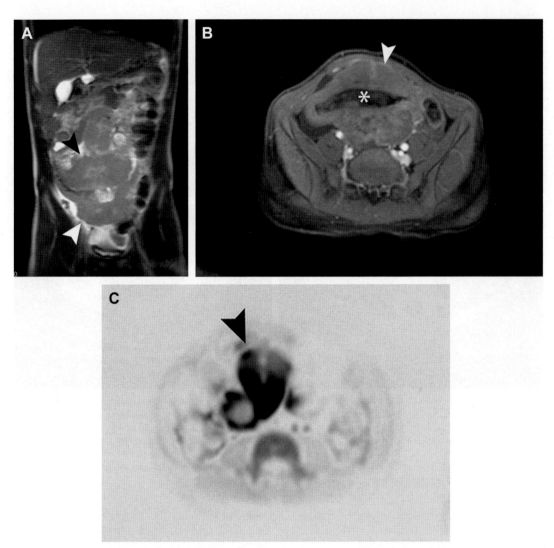

Fig. 3. Burkitt lymphoma in a 7-year-old boy. (*A*) Coronal T2-weighted image demonstrates intermediate-signal mass (*arrowheads*) on either side of the bowel lumen. A small amount of ascites is also present. (*B*) Axial T1-weighted image with fat saturation following intravenous gadolinium chelate reveals the minimally enhancing mass thickening the bowel wall (*arrowhead*) and aneurysmal dilation of the lumen (*asterisk*). (*C*) Axial inverted diffusion-weighted image shows restricted diffusion in the thickened bowel wall (*arrowhead*).

situation requires urgent steroid treatment to shrink the tumor; however, steroids cause so rapid a response that a tissue specimen obtained subsequently may not be adequate for diagnosis. Consequently, tissue for diagnosis, as well as imaging for staging, is best obtained before administration of steroids. Yet, the respiratory distress may preclude sedation and even supine positioning in a scanner. CT may be possible with the head elevated to 30° and with critical care specialists in attendance. If blasts are present in peripheral blood or in pleural fluid, then a diagnosis can be obtained without biopsy of the mediastinal mass. If necessary, the mass may be sampled

with the patient in an upright position using ultrasound guidance and local anesthesia.[23,24]

Pathology Findings

Pathology examination reveals a proliferation of small-sized to intermediate-sized cells with scant cytoplasm, small nucleoli, and fine chromatin. Tingible body macrophages with ingested apoptotic debris are scattered among these cells, conferring a starry-sky appearance similar to that seen in Burkitt lymphoma.[7,13] Necrosis may be noted along with increased mitotic rate.[13] Almost all lymphoblastic lymphomas are derived from T-cell

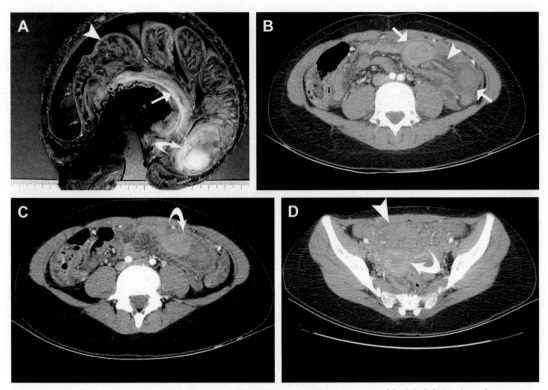

Fig. 4. Burkitt lymphoma causing enteroenteric intussusception in a 15-year-old girl. (*A*) Sectioned gross specimen reveals small bowel loops (*arrowhead*) within a loop of small bowel. Mesenteric fat is also noted (*arrow*). The white circumscribed lead point mass is demonstrated (*curved arrow*). (*B*) Axial CT image shows the concentric ring appearance of bowel within bowel of an intussusception (*arrow*) with mesenteric fat of the intussusceptum in the center (*arrowhead*). (*C*) Axial CT image obtained cephalad to (*B*) reveals the mildly enhancing lead-point mass (*curved arrow*). (*D*) Axial CT image of the pelvis demonstrates soft tissue attenuation (*arrowhead*) anterior to the uterus (*curved arrow*) representing omental caking.

lineage and the immunophenotype of lymphoblastic lymphoma is that of an immature T-cell (CD3, CD4, CD5, and CD7 positivity).[7,13]

Imaging Features

Anterior mediastinal mass is the most frequent finding (70%–75% of patients). The mediastinal mass is caused by diffuse infiltration of the thymus, so the appearance is of diffuse enlargement rather than the heterogeneous nodular appearance that characterizes Hodgkin lymphoma or other forms of NHL (**Fig. 10**). Nodal and other extranodal sites may also be affected, particularly cervical and supraclavicular nodes.[2,25] Pleural and pericardial effusion are also common findings (see **Fig. 10**).[2,13] Renal involvement is not unusual and manifests as organ enlargement with hypoattenuating cortical masses (**Fig. 11**).[2] Other sites of involvement include liver, spleen, lung, CNS, bone marrow, and testes; however, these are usually involved in conjunction with the anterior mediastinum (**Figs. 12** and **13**). Unlike other forms of pediatric NHL, CNS involvement is

relatively common in lymphoblastic lymphoma and CNS prophylaxis is administered to all patients.[2] Bone and soft tissue involvement may also be seen.

DIFFUSE LARGE B-CELL LYMPHOMA

DLBCL constitutes 20% of childhood lymphomas and is the most common type of NHL affecting children with congenital or acquired immunodeficiency.[2,13] The disease is slightly more common in male patients.[7] The incidence increases with advancing age and is uncommon in children younger than age 5 years.[1] Only 2 subtypes are observed in children: primary mediastinal large B-cell lymphoma (PMBL) and disseminated disease. Patients most often present with the disseminated form.[26] PMBL is more common in adolescents and is associated with a better prognosis than the disseminated form.[27] Low-stage disease at presentation is seen in almost half of patients with DLBCL.[7] Peripheral adenopathy is common.

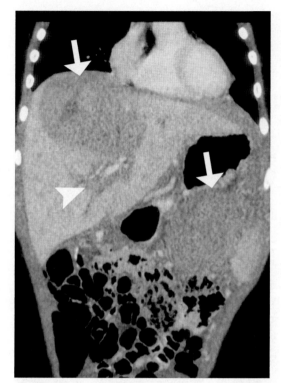

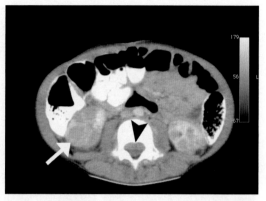

Fig. 7. CT following intravenous iodinated contrast shows multiple cortically-based hypoattenuating masses of the kidneys (*arrow*). Additionally, there is abnormal enhancing tissue in the spinal canal (*arrowhead*).

Fig. 5. Burkitt lymphoma in an 8-year-old boy. Coronal contrast-enhanced CT demonstrates hypoattenuating masses in the liver and mesentery (*arrows*). Hypoattenuating tissue around the portal vein is noted consistent with tumor infiltration (*arrowhead*).

Pathology Findings

Fibrosis intermixed with tumor cells is common, particularly in the mediastinum. Tumor cells are medium-sized to large lymphoid cells with abundant amphophilic or densely eosinophilic cytoplasm.[13] Often the tumor is polymorphic, also containing pleomorphic cells that may appear polylobate or even frankly anaplastic. The tumor cells stain positively with pan B-cell markers (CD19, CD20, CD22, and CD79a).[7,13]

Imaging Features

Patients present with extranodal disease in up to 40% of cases.[7] PMBL appears similar to Hodgkin lymphoma on imaging (**Fig. 14**), whereas the more frequent disseminated form of DLBCL most often involves the GI tract and mimics Burkitt lymphoma (**Fig. 15**). The presence of peripheral adenopathy and or immunodeficiency suggests DLBCL instead of Hodgkin and Burkitt lymphoma.[2] Similarly, cortical bone involvement is more in keeping with DLBCL than Burkitt lymphoma. Other common sites of involvement with focal masses include liver, spleen, and kidney, similar to Burkitt

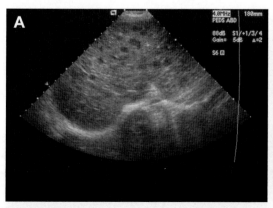

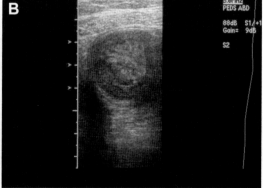

Fig. 6. Burkitt lymphoma in an 11-year-old girl after renal transplant. (*A*) Transverse ultrasound of the liver demonstrates multiple small hypoechoic lesions in the liver. (*B*) Ultrasound of the right lower quadrant reveals the doughnut sign of intussusception.

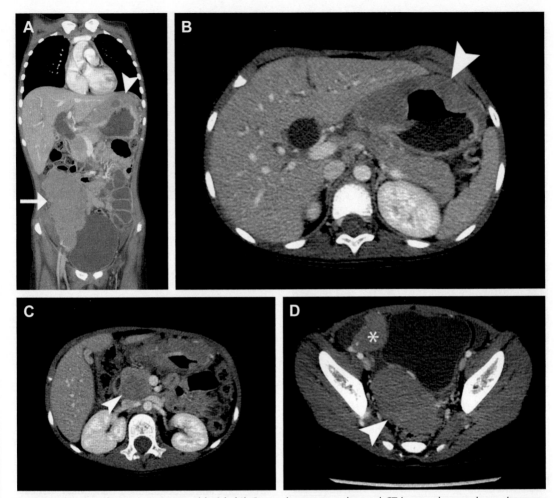

Fig. 8. Burkitt lymphoma in a 9-year-old girl. (*A*) Coronal contrast-enhanced CT image shows a large, homogeneous right lower quadrant (pelvic) mass involving the right ovary (*arrow*). Also noted is marked thickening of the stomach wall (*arrowhead*). (*B*) Axial CT image shows the thickened wall of the stomach (*arrowhead*). (*C*) Axial CT image obtained caudal to (*B*) shows a retroperitoneal mass (*arrowhead*) adjacent to the superior mesenteric vein. (*D*) Axial CT image through the pelvis shows an enlarged left ovary (*arrowhead*). Asterisk indicates the right lower quadrant mass seen in (*A*).

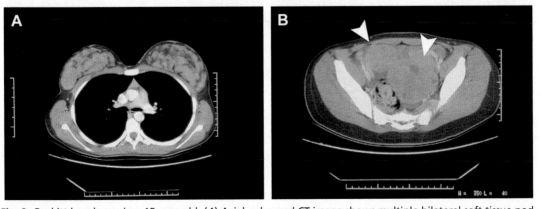

Fig. 9. Burkitt lymphoma in a 15-year-old. (*A*) Axial enhanced CT image shows multiple bilateral soft tissue nodules in both breasts. (*B*) Axial image through the pelvis reveals involvement of the bilateral ovaries (*arrowheads*).

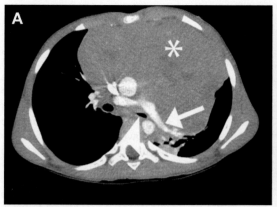
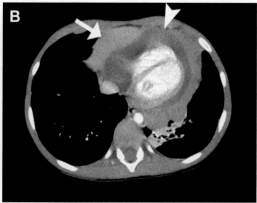

Fig. 10. Six-year-old boy with acute T-cell lymphoblastic leukemia. (*A*) Axial CT following intravenous contrast reveals a large homogeneous anterior mediastinal mass (*asterisk*) causing compression of the pulmonary arteries (*arrow*) and the left mainstem bronchus (*arrowhead*). (*B*) Axial CT image obtained caudal to (*A*) shows the anterior mediastinal mass (*arrow*) and a large pericardial effusion (*arrowhead*).

lymphoma (**Figs. 16** and **17**). Mesenteric and retroperitoneal lymphadenopathy may also be seen.

Additional sites of disease include salivary glands, Waldeyer ring, thyroid, adrenal gland, and testes.[7] Bone marrow is involved in 11% to 27% of cases.[7] Malignant pericardial and pleural effusions, as well as lung involvement, may also be seen (see **Fig. 14**).

ANAPLASTIC LARGE CELL LYMPHOMA

ALCL is a mature T-cell lymphoma that accounts for 10% to 15% of NHL in children.[13,28] The mean age in children is 10 years and the tumor is far more common in male patients.[2,28] ALCL

involves both nodal and extranodal sites. Most children present with advanced stage disease. B symptoms (fever, night sweats, and weight loss) are common (75%), particularly fever.[7,13]

Pathology Findings

The tumors cells are very large with abundant eosinophilic cytoplasm. These often contain wreath-shaped or horseshoe-shaped nuclei with an eosinophilic region near the nucleus. Such cells are termed hallmark cells because they are present in all histologic variants of ALCL.[7,13] In contrast to adults, almost all pediatric tumors demonstrate the t(2:5) translocation involving the anaplastic lymphoma kinase (ALK) oncogene, and 95% react positively to antibodies against

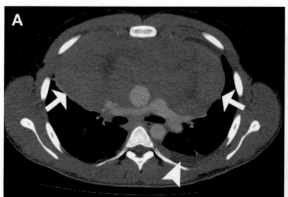
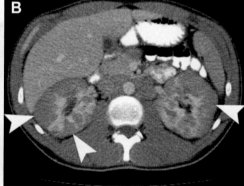

Fig. 11. T-cell lymphoblastic lymphoma in a 19-year-old boy. (*A*) Axial CT image following intravenous contrast shows a large, relatively homogeneous anterior mediastinal mass (*arrows*) and a left pleural effusion (*arrowhead*). (*B*) Axial CT image of the upper abdomen shows multiple peripheral hypoattenuating masses of the kidneys (*arrowheads*).

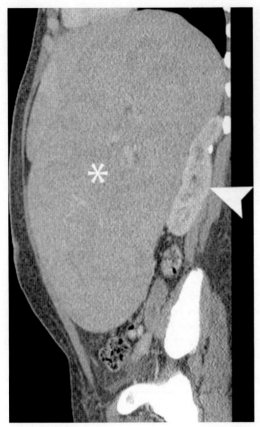

Fig. 12. T-cell lymphoblastic lymphoma in a child showing marked homogeneous enlargement of the spleen (*asterisk*) causing compression of the left kidney (*arrowhead*).

the ALK gene product.[7,13,28] All tumor cells demonstrate staining for CD30 in the cell membrane and Golgi region. Tumors cells also stain positively for some T-cell markers and epithelial membrane antigen.[7,13]

Imaging Features

Mediastinal masses are common in ALCL.[29] Extranodal sites of involvement include lung, liver, bone, soft tissue, and skin (**Figs. 18** and **19**).[7,25,28] Bone disease may mimic a primary bone tumor and the finding of additional sites of disease is helpful in suggesting the proper diagnosis. Lung disease may appear as multiple nodules with ill-defined borders and possibly cavitation or dense consolidation mimicking pneumonia similar to other forms of NHL. A reticulonodular pattern due to compression by a mediastinal mass or adenopathy may also be seen.[23] A mediastinal mass is found in less than half of patients.[25] Large malignant pleural or pericardial effusions are frequently seen. Cervical and retroperitoneal lymph nodes may be involved. Incidence of bone marrow involvement depends on method of diagnosis and is as high as 30% when immunohistochemical staining for CD30 and ALK is used.[28] Detection is even higher if molecular studies are applied.[28] CNS disease is rare.[2,28]

APPROACH TO IMAGING DIAGNOSIS AND STAGING OF NON-HODGKIN LYMPHOMA

Treatment is risk-adapted based on initial disease staging. Advances in imaging technology over the past several decades have allowed imaging to replace surgical staging of lymphoma. Pediatric NHL tends to involve the chest or the abdomen. The mediastinal mass is often initially discovered on chest radiograph obtained for respiratory symptoms and abdominal masses found on ultrasound obtained for abdominal pain. Ultrasound is also valuable in the assessment of testicular disease.

Generally, CT of the chest, abdomen, and pelvis with oral and intravenous contrast media is the

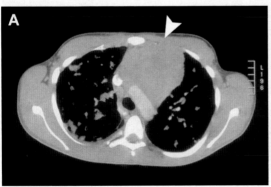
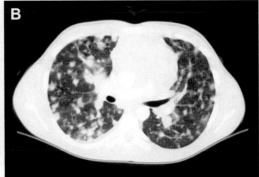

Fig. 13. B-cell lymphoblastic lymphoma in a 16-year-old boy. (*A*) Axial contrast-enhanced CT shows a homogeneous mediastinal mass (*arrowhead*) and numerous lung nodules. (*B*) Axial CT image in lung windows better depicts the diffuse lung nodules.

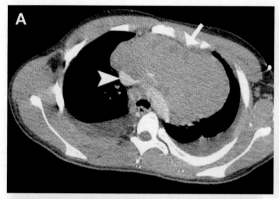

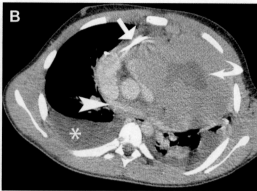

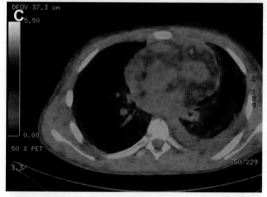

Fig. 14. DLBCL in a 16-year-old boy. (*A*) Axial contrast-enhanced CT image shows a large homogeneous anterior mediastinal mass (*arrow*) causing compression of the superior vena cava (*arrowhead*). (*B*) Axial CT image obtained caudal to (*A*) shows a central low attenuation focus (*curved arrow*) within the mediastinal mass consistent with necrosis. The mass compresses the left atrium (*arrowhead*). Pleural effusion (*asterisk*) is noted bilaterally and a pericardial drain is seen (*arrow*). (*C*) Fused image from FDG-PET/CT reveals uptake of radiotracer within the anterior mediastinal mass.

most commonly used study for initial disease staging, more recently in conjunction with fluorodeoxyglucose (FDG)-PET. Age-appropriate and size-appropriate dosing and single-phase imaging should be used to minimize radiation dose in children in accordance with the as low as reasonably achievable (ALARA) principle. CT of the neck is performed if there is palpable cervical adenopathy or concern for involvement of the parapharyngeal lymphoid (Waldeyer) ring.[18]

Due to concerns about cumulative ionizing radiation dose, MR imaging can be considered as an alternative to CT imaging, although PET data is more readily obtained in conjunction with diagnostic CT owing to the increasing availability of integrated PET/CT systems. MR imaging is superior for evaluation for CNS disease; however, CNS involvement is rare, so MR imaging of the brain is pursued only if there are suggestive clinical signs.[2,18] MR imaging is also useful for evaluation of focal bone involvement, and whole-body (WB) MR imaging has been shown to be more sensitive for evaluation of bone marrow disease than bone scintigraphy.[30,31] MR imaging is inferior to CT imaging for the evaluation of disease involving the lung.[31,32]

^{18}F-FDG PET and hybrid ^{18}F-FDG PET fused with diagnostic CT have replaced gallium (^{67}Ga) and bone scintigraphy for disease staging. Most of the subtypes of lymphoma that affect children are aggressive and show strong FDG-avidity.[33–35] Compared with gallium scan, FDG-PET scanning delivers a lower radiation dose with improved spatial resolution and imaging can be performed on the same day the radiopharmaceutical is administered. Studies in adults and children with NHL showed improved sensitivity and specificity in the assessment of stage using FDG-PET and FDG-PET/CT compared with gallium scanning, bone scan, and conventional cross-sectional imaging studies.[26,36–42] Furthermore, FDG-PET/CT has been shown to alter staging, resulting in a modification of treatment in up to one-third of patients.[10,26,36,39–43] The sensitivity and specificity of PET/CT for lymphoma staging in children are 96% to 99%, and 95% to 100%, respectively.[44]

The St. Jude (Murphy) staging system (**Table 1**), developed more than 3 decades ago, has traditionally been applied to all types of NHL. Stage I and II disease is considered

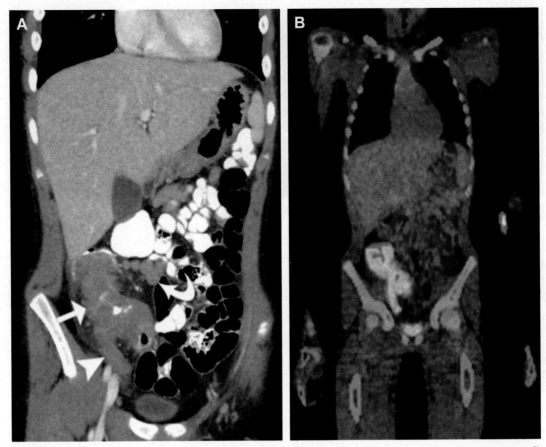

Fig. 15. DLBCL in a 12-year-old boy. (*A*) Coronal CT scan following intravenous and oral contrast media administration reveals marked mural thickening of the terminal ileum and cecum (*arrow*) as well as the appendix (*arrowhead*). Mild surrounding inflammatory change and enlarged regional lymph nodes (*arrowhead*) are noted. (*B*) Coronal fused FDG-PET/CT image shows marked tracer uptake at the sites of bowel wall thickening.

localized, whereas stage III and IV disease is disseminated, requiring aggressive combination chemotherapy. There are several limitations of this system, including lack of inclusion of many extranodal sites of disease that are more common in children and lack of consideration of findings of newer more advanced modalities of disease detection.[22] Recently, a revised international staging system (International Pediatric NHL Staging System [IPNHLSS]) has been developed to facilitate more accurate staging and comparison of efficacy for studies of treatment strategies (**Table 2**).[22]

ASSESSMENT OF RESPONSE TO THERAPY

The 5-year survival rate for NHL is now 76% to 85%, and is better for younger children compared with adolescents.[1,45,46] Patients with refractory or relapsed disease fare far worse than patients with early response, so the goal of therapy is to obtain early complete remission using aggressive chemotherapy protocols.[25] Detection of early response or lack thereof allows early modification of therapy to increase the chance of complete remission in poor responders and spare those with good response from unnecessary treatment-related toxicities.[25,43] Because metabolic response to therapy precedes change in size of the tumor mass, FDG-PET imaging has been shown to be more accurate for the detection of early response to therapy than imaging based on conventional size; therefore it can be used to modify therapy.[34,38,39,42,43,47] Furthermore, because tumors often contain fibrotic tissue that may remain after active tumor has been destroyed, FDG-PET has been shown to have superior negative predictive value for residual

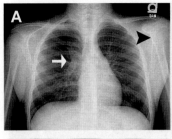

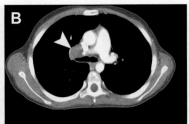

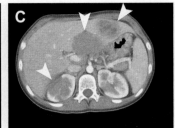

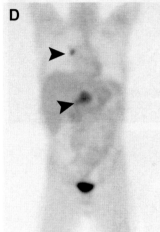

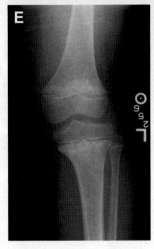

Fig. 16. DLBCL in a 12-year-old boy with McKusick type metaphyseal chondrodysplasia, which is associated with congenital immune deficiency. (*A*) Chest radiograph shows right hilar enlargement (*arrow*) and a fracture of the left humeral neck (*arrowhead*). (*B*) Contrast-enhanced CT image shows right hilar adenopathy (*arrowhead*). (*C*) CT image demonstrates hypoattenuating masses of the liver and kidneys (*arrowheads*). (*D*) Coronal FDG-PET SPECT image demonstrates radiotracer uptake in the right hilum and the liver lesion (*arrowheads*). Uptake was also seen in the kidneys and the left shoulder (not shown). (*E*) Radiograph of the knee reveals irregular metaphyses from underlying metaphyseal chondrodysplasia.

disease after completion of therapy compared with conventional imaging,[42,48–50] although further study is required to confirm this finding in children.[32]

The specificity of FDG-PET is hampered by several sources of false positive results, including metabolically active brown fat, muscle, infection, inflammation, radiation pneumonitis, bone marrow conversion, and spleen activity induced by granulocyte-stimulating factor.[26,33,48,51,52] False positives are reduced by correlation with CT or MR imaging findings or with close interval follow-up imaging.[23]

Rebound thymic hyperplasia is a well-established phenomenon that mimics mediastinal tumor recurrence. The process typically peaks 6 to 12 months following completion of therapy but may occur as early as 1 week later.[18,53,54] The normal thymus changes in size and appearance with age. The thymus in infants and young children is quadrilateral in configuration with convex margins and homogeneous in appearance (**Fig. 20**). With advancing age, the thymus changes to a triangular shape with concave margins. The gland becomes more heterogeneous in appearance as fat replaces the gland (**Fig. 21**). The normal thymus

is soft and does not compress or displace mediastinal vessels. Thymic rebound appears on FDG-PET and CT imaging as an enlarged bilobed homogeneous gland with mild, diffuse uptake of FDG. Imaging follow-up is preferred to biopsy in these cases (**Fig. 22**).[25] On the other hand, if the standardized uptake value (SUV) is 3.4 or higher, relapsed disease is more likely and biopsy is indicated.[55]

The same response criteria are used for interim assessment and for restaging at completion of therapy. The International Harmonization Project (IHP) was recently convened to revise and unify the response criteria for adults to include functional and metabolic data as well as more recent outcomes data to create the new Laguno response classification system. However, data from scientific studies in children were not considered in creating this system and the histologic spectrum of NHL that affects children is unique.[56] For these reasons, a new set of response criteria based on the IHP criteria for adults has been proposed for the pediatric population.[32] The investigators emphasize that the use of FDG-PET data in clinical decision-making in children is still considered

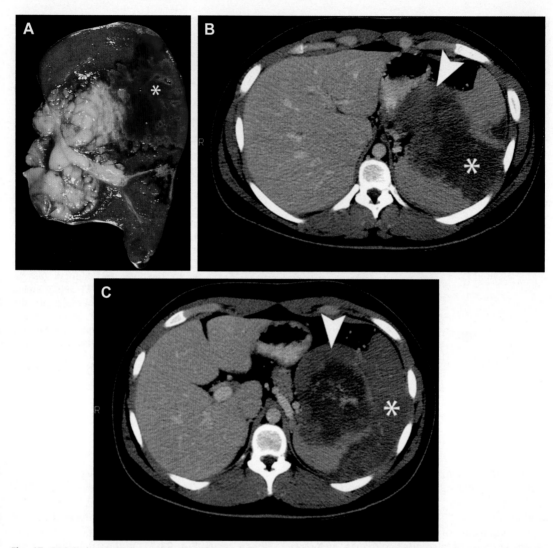

Fig. 17. DLBCL in an 18-year-old patient with left upper quadrant pain after a martial arts class. (*A*) Photograph of sectioned gross specimen shows a lobulated whitish mass and contiguous laceration (*asterisk*). (*B*) Axial contrast-enhanced CT image reveals a hypoattenuating splenic mass (*arrowhead*) and adjacent wide linear laceration (*asterisk*). (*C*) Axial CT image obtained caudal to (*B*) shows the mass (*arrowhead*) with some central high attenuation consistent with active bleeding. Adjacent subcapsular hemorrhage is noted (*asterisk*).

investigational and should be limited to the context of a clinical trial.[32] They also recommend that FDG-PET activity in the tumor be measured based on a reproducible scale such as the Deauville scale (uptake is compared with that of the mediastinal blood pool and liver or spleen)[57] or change in maximum SUV.[32]

RELAPSE SURVEILLANCE

Imaging is used for relapse surveillance; however, patients with lymphoma receive a considerable cumulative radiation dose, and the benefit of frequent and prolonged routine imaging surveillance several years after therapy completion has recently been questioned.[23,58,59] Relapses are rare after complete remission. Most occur within the first year after completion of therapy and are generally suspected on clinical grounds.[23,59]

COMPLICATIONS OF THERAPY

With aggressive multiagent chemotherapy regimens, overall survival is good and the goal of future improvements in therapy is shifting

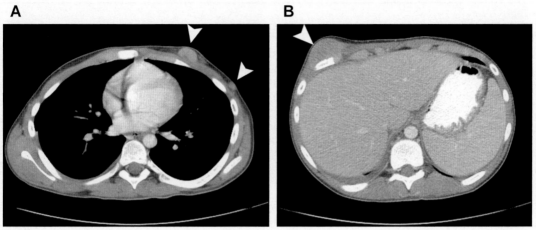

Fig. 18. ALCL in a 16-year-old boy. (*A*) Axial CT after intravenous contrast shows 2 small subcutaneous masses (*arrowheads*). (*B*) CT image obtained caudal to (*B*) shows a larger mass in the muscle and the chest wall (*arrowhead*).

toward reduction of complications. Short-term complications include tumor lysis syndrome (characteristic of Burkitt lymphoma), atypical and opportunistic infections, neutropenic enterocolitis (typhlitis), methotrexate leukoencephalopathy, posterior reversible encephalopathy syndrome, deep venous thrombosis, hepatic venoocclusive disease, and graft-versus-host disease. Late complications include respiratory compromise due to bleomycin or radiation therapy, cardiac compromise due to anthracyclines or radiation therapy, osteoporosis and osteonecrosis related to steroid or radiation therapy, post-transplant lymphoproliferative disorder, and secondary malignancy. The risk of

secondary malignancy is well known and greater in patients who are younger at time of diagnosis.[2,7] The risk with newer low-dose radiation therapy regimens is not clear. The latency period may be longer for lower dose therapy.[25]

Table 1 St. Jude staging system	
Stage I	Single tumor with exclusion of mediastinum and abdomen
Stage II	Single EN tumor with regional lymph node involvement ≥2 EN tumors or N areas of involvement on the same side of the diaphragm Primary GI tract tumor with or without regional lymph node involvement only, completely resected
Stage III	≥2 EN tumors or areas of nodal involvement on opposite sides of the diaphragm Primary intrathoracic tumor Extensive primary intraabdominal disease, not resectable Paraspinal or epidural tumor
Stage IV	Findings of any of stages I-III with CNS or bone involvement at presentation

Abbreviations: EN, extranodal; N, nodal.

Data from Murphy S. Childhood non-Hodgkin's lymphoma. N Engl J Med 1978;299:1446–8.

Fig. 19. ALCL. Axial CT shows a large chest wall mass (*arrow*) extending into the pleural space. Enlarged mediastinal nodes (*arrowhead*) are seen, as well as left upper lobe atelectasis.

Table 2
International Pediatric Non-Hodgkin Lymphoma Staging System

Stage I	Single tumor with exclusion of mediastinum and abdomen
Stage II	Single EN tumor with regional node involvement $\geq$ 2 N areas of same side of diaphragm Primary GI tract tumor, +/− involvement of associated mesenteric nodes that is completely resectable
Stage III	$\geq$ 2 EN tumors above and below diaphragm $\geq$ 2 N areas above and below diaphragm Intrathoracic tumor Intraabdominal and retroperitoneal disease (except primary GI tract tumor as described in Stage II) Paraspinal or epidural tumor Single B lesion with concomitant involvement of EN and/or non-regional N sites
Stage IV	Any of the above findings with initial involvement of CNS, BM or both on conventional methods

Abbreviations: B, bone; BM, bone marrow; EN, extranodal; N, nodal.
Data from Rosolen A, Perkins SL, Pinkerton CR, et al. Revised International Pediatric Non-Hodgkin Lymphoma Staging System. J Clin Onc 2015;33(18):2112–8.

FUTURE DIRECTIONS

WB MR imaging with short tau inversion-recovery (STIR) with or without other sequences is being explored as an alternative to PET/CT without the risk of ionizing radiation. Limitations include loss of resolution with large field of view and long scan times. In younger patients, the risk of sedation must also be weighed against the risks of exposure to ionizing radiation.[60,61] Recent advances in techniques, including phased-array and multichannel coils, as well as parallel imaging,

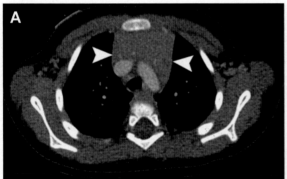

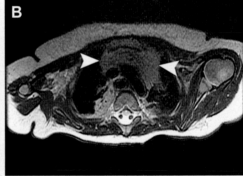

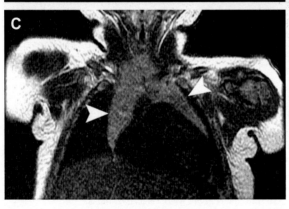

Fig. 20. Normal thymus in an infant. (*A*) Axial CT in a 14-month-old girl shows a homogeneous structure of similar attenuation to muscle (*arrowheads*). Note the quadrilateral configuration and slightly convex margins. (*B*) Axial T2-weighted image of the same girl at age 6 months shows that the thymus is of homogeneous intermediate signal intensity (*arrowheads*) with convex margins (*arrowheads*). Note the thymus does not compress the vessels. Medial atelectasis is seen related to sedation. (*C*) Coronal T2-weighted image shows the homogeneous thymus (*arrowheads*) with a bilobed configuration draped over the heart.

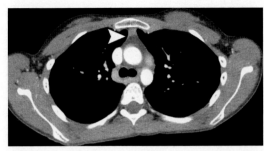

Fig. 21. CT image of normal thymus in a 16-year-old girl demonstrates the triangular configuration with a mixture of fat and soft tissue attenuation (*arrowhead*).

have reduced scan times to the range of those of other WB imaging studies.[62] Additionally, the development of respiratory gating and triggering, balanced steady-state imaging, and motion correction sequences have allowed reduction of motion artifact.[62]

WB MR imaging has been shown to have good agreement with PET/CT in the staging of pediatric lymphoma.[30,63] On the other hand, a recent multi-center prospective trial by Siegel and colleagues[31] did not demonstrate noninferiority of WB MR imaging compared with a combination of techniques other than FDG-PET for staging, particularly for disease of the lung and solid organs. The investigators concluded that WB MR imaging should not be used as the sole imaging modality.

WB diffusion-weighted (DW) imaging also shows promise for evaluation of children with lymphoma. Lymphoma is highly cellular with high nuclear-to-cytoplasmic ratios and most lymphomas show diffusion restriction. Early studies show high correlation with PET/CT.[64–66] WB DW

imaging with background signal suppression allows imaging with free breathing and has been recently shown to provide comparable detection of malignant adenopathy and extranodal disease in malignant lymphomas compared with FDG-PET/CT.[67]

WB diffusion does have some limitations. Normal lymph nodes are also densely cellular and show diffusion restriction. Studies of apparent diffusion coefficient (ADC) measurements undertaken to determine if lymphomatous nodes can be distinguished from uninvolved nodes based on ADC values have shown mixed results.[62,64,68] In addition, DWI is not specific for malignant tumor because some normal tissues also demonstrate restricted diffusion, including red bone marrow, thymus, spleen, adrenal glands, salivary glands, and gonads.[62] Changes in diffusion characteristics may allow assessment of tumor response to therapy because initial studies have shown increase in ADC values after successful chemotherapy in pediatric lymphoma, and diffusion and ADC values may be useful in conjunction with FDG-PET data to predict interim response.[62,63,66,69]

A limitation of all anatomic imaging is false negative results due to involvement of normal-sized lymph nodes, liver, and spleen. The new technology of integrated PET/MR has likely overcome this limitation with reduced radiation exposure compared with PET/CT. A recent study reported a radiation dose reduction of 80%.[70] When combined with WB DW imaging, a PET/MR examination can be completed within 60 minutes, similar to FDG-PET/CT. In addition, PET/MR affords the advantage of higher soft tissue resolution and better definition of tumor anatomy, along with information about perfusion and diffusion.

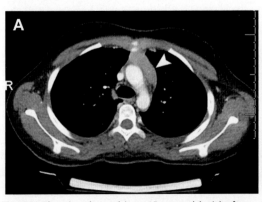
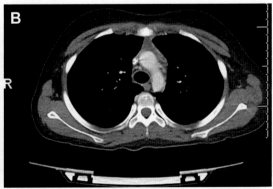

Fig. 22. Thymic rebound in a 13-year-old girl after completion of therapy for lymphoma with history of large mediastinal mass. (*A*) Initial post-therapy CT image with intravenous contrast shows a homogeneous soft tissue mass in the anterior mediastinum with convex margins (*arrowhead*). (*B*) Follow-up CT demonstrates normal triangular configuration and lower (fat) attenuation of the thymus.

SUMMARY

In summary, compared with adult disease, pediatric extranodal lymphoma has a far more limited histologic spectrum with preponderance of aggressive subtypes presenting with widespread disease. In addition, children are more susceptible to long-term effects of the significant cumulative radiation dose delivered to oncologic patients, a concern that is driving the study of alternative imaging techniques for staging and follow-up.

REFERENCES

1. Percy CL, Smith MA, Linet M, et al. Lymphomas and reticuloendothelial neoplasms. In: Ries LAG, Smith MA, Gurney JG, et al, editors. Cancer incidence and survival among children and adolescents: United States SEER Program. Bethesda (MD): NIH; 1999. p. 35–50.

2. Abramson SJ, Price AP. Imaging of pediatric lymphomas. Radiol Clin North Am 2008;46(2): 313–38, ix.

3. Mbulaiteye SM, Anderson WF, Bhatia K, et al. Trimodal age-specific incidence patterns for Burkitt lymphoma in the United States, 1973-2005. Int J Cancer 2010;126(7):1732–9.

4. Biko DM, Anupindi SA, Hernandez A, et al. Childhood Burkitt lymphoma: abdominal and pelvic imaging findings. AJR Am J Roentgenol 2009;192(5): 1304–15.

5. Feller AC, Diebold J. Histopathology of nodal and extranodal non-Hodgkin's lymphoma. Berlin: Springer-Verlag; 2004.

6. Stovroff MC, Coran AG, Hutchinson RJ. The role of surgery in American Burkitt's lymphoma in children. J Pediatr Surg 1991;26(10):1235–8.

7. Swerdlow SH, Campo E, Harris NL, et al. WHO classification of tumours of haematopoietic and lymphoid tissues. 4th edition. Lyon (France): International Agency for Research on Cancer; 2009.

8. Brady G, MacArthur GJ, Farrell PJ. Epstein-Barr virus and Burkitt lymphoma. J Clin Pathol 2007; 60(12):1397–402.

9. Molyneux EM, Rochford R, Griffin B, et al. Burkitt's lymphoma. Lancet 2012;379(9822):1234–44.

10. Cheng G, Chen W, Chamroonrat W, et al. Biopsy versus FDG PET/CT in the initial evaluation of bone marrow involvement in pediatric lymphoma patients. Eur J Nucl Med Mol Imaging 2011;38(8):1469–76.

11. Kamona AA, El-Khatib MA, Swaidan MY, et al. Pediatric Burkitt's lymphoma: CT findings. Abdom Imaging 2007;32(3):381–6.

12. Hecht JL, Aster JC. Molecular biology of Burkitt's lymphoma. J Clin Oncol 2000;18(21):3707–21.

13. McCurley TL, Zutter MM, Sheehan AM. The lymph nodes, spleen, and thymus. In: Stocker JT, Dehner LP, Husain AN, editors. Stocker and dehner's pediatric pathology. 3rd edition. Philadelphia: Lippincott Williams & Wilkins; 2010. p. 975–1009.

14. Ghai S, Pattison J, Ghai S, et al. Primary gastrointestinal lymphoma: spectrum of imaging findings with pathologic correlation. Radiographics 2007;27(5): 1371–88.

15. Chung EM, Biko DM, Arzamendi AM, et al. Solid tumors of the peritoneum, omentum, and mesentery in children: radiologic-pathologic correlation: from the radiologic pathology archives. Radiographics 2015;35(2):521–46.

16. Gollub MJ. Imaging of gastrointestinal lymphoma. Radiol Clin North Am 2008;46(2):287–312, ix.

17. Vade A, Blane CE. Imaging of Burkitt lymphoma in pediatric patients. Pediatr Radiol 1985;15(2): 123–6.

18. Toma P, Granata C, Rossi A, et al. Multimodality imaging of Hodgkin disease and non-Hodgkin lymphomas in children. Radiographics 2007;27(5): 1335–54.

19. Seltzer SE, Jochelson M, Balikian JP. Organ envelopment in lymphoma visualised by computed tomography. Clin Radiol 1986;37(6): 525–9.

20. Leite NP, Kased N, Hanna RF, et al. Cross-sectional imaging of extranodal involvement in abdominopelvic lymphoproliferative malignancies. Radiographics 2007;27(6):1613–34.

21. Goodman P, Raval B. Omental cakes in American Burkitt lymphoma. Computed tomography demonstration. Clin Imaging 1989;13(2):117–8.

22. Rosolen A, Perkins SL, Pinkerton CR, et al. Revised International Pediatric Non-Hodgkin Lymphoma Staging System. J Clin Oncol 2015; 33(18):2112–8.

23. Averill LW, Acikgoz G, Miller RE, et al. Update on pediatric leukemia and lymphoma imaging. Semin Ultrasound CT MR 2013;34(6):578–99.

24. Perger L, Lee EY, Shamberger RC. Management of children and adolescents with a critical airway due to compression by an anterior mediastinal mass. J Pediatr Surg 2008;43(11):1990–7.

25. Guillerman RP, Voss SD, Parker BR. Leukemia and lymphoma. Radiol Clin North Am 2011; 49(4):767–97, vii.

26. Furth C, Denecke T, Steffen I, et al. Correlative imaging strategies implementing CT, MRI, and PET for staging of childhood Hodgkin disease. J Pediatr Hematol Oncol 2006;28(8):501–12.

27. Nagle SJ, Chong EA, Chekol S, et al. The role of FDG-PET imaging as a prognostic marker of outcome in primary mediastinal B-cell lymphoma. Cancer Med 2015;4(1):7–15.

28. Lowe EJ, Gross TG. Anaplastic large cell lymphoma in children and adolescents. Pediatr Hematol Oncol 2013;30(6):509–19.

29. Williams DM, Hobson R, Imeson J, et al. Anaplastic large cell lymphoma in childhood: analysis of 72 patients treated on The United Kingdom Children's Cancer Study Group chemotherapy regimens. Br J Haematol 2002;117(4):812–20.

30. Kellenberger CJ, Miller SF, Khan M, et al. Initial experience with FSE STIR whole-body MR imaging for staging lymphoma in children. Eur Radiol 2004; 14(10):1829–41.

31. Siegel MJ, Acharyya S, Hoffer FA, et al. Whole-body MR imaging for staging of malignant tumors in pediatric patients: results of the American College of Radiology Imaging Network 6660 Trial. Radiology 2013;266(2):599–609.

32. Sandlund JT, Guillerman RP, Perkins SL, et al. International Pediatric Non-Hodgkin Lymphoma Response Criteria. J Clin Oncol 2015;33(18):2106–11.

33. Bardi E, Csoka M, Garai I, et al. Value of FDG-PET/CT examinations in different cancers of children, focusing on lymphomas. Pathol Oncol Res 2014; 20(1):139–43.

34. Karantanis D, Durski JM, Lowe VJ, et al. 18F-FDG PET and PET/CT in Burkitt's lymphoma. Eur J Radiol 2010;75(1):e68–73.

35. Seam P, Juweid ME, Cheson BD. The role of FDG-PET scans in patients with lymphoma. Blood 2007; 110(10):3507–16.

36. Depas G, De Barsy C, Jerusalem G, et al. 18F-FDG PET in children with lymphomas. Eur J Nucl Med Mol Imaging 2005;32(1):31–8.

37. Edeline V, Bonardel G, Brisse H, et al. Prospective study of 18F-FDG PET in pediatric mediastinal lymphoma: a single center experience. Leuk Lymphoma 2007;48(4):823–6.

38. London K, Cross S, Onikul E, et al. 18F-FDG PET/CT in paediatric lymphoma: comparison with conventional imaging. Eur J Nucl Med Mol Imaging 2011; 38(2):274–84.

39. Miller E, Metser U, Avrahami G, et al. Role of 18F-FDG PET/CT in staging and follow-up of lymphoma in pediatric and young adult patients. J Comput Assist Tomogr 2006;30(4):689–94.

40. Montravers F, McNamara D, Landman-Parker J, et al. [(18)F]FDG in childhood lymphoma: clinical utility and impact on management. Eur J Nucl Med Mol Imaging 2002;29(9):1155–65.

41. Riad R, Omar W, Kotb M, et al. Role of PET/CT in malignant pediatric lymphoma. Eur J Nucl Med Mol Imaging 2010;37(2):319–29.

42. Mody RJ, Bui C, Hutchinson RJ, et al. Comparison of (18)F Flurodeoxyglucose PET with Ga-67 scintigraphy and conventional imaging modalities in pediatric lymphoma. Leuk Lymphoma 2007;48(4): 699–707.

43. Freebody J, Wegner EA, Rossleigh MA. 2-deoxy-2-((18)F)fluoro-D-glucose positron emission tomography/computed tomography imaging in paediatric oncology. World J Radiol 2014;6(10): 741–55.

44. Uslu L, Donig J, Link M, et al. Value of 18F-FDG PET and PET/CT for evaluation of pediatric malignancies. J Nucl Med 2015;56(2):274–86.

45. Smith MA, Seibel NL, Altekruse SF, et al. Outcomes for children and adolescents with cancer: challenges for the twenty-first century. J Clin Oncol 2010;28(15):2625–34.

46. Ward E, DeSantis C, Robbins A, et al. Childhood and adolescent cancer statistics, 2014. CA Cancer J Clin 2014;64(2):83–103.

47. Kluge R, Kurch L, Montravers F, et al. FDG PET/CT in children and adolescents with lymphoma. Pediatr Radiol 2013;43(4):406–17.

48. Bhojwani D, McCarville MB, Choi JK, et al. The role of FDG-PET/CT in the evaluation of residual disease in paediatric non-Hodgkin lymphoma. Br J Haematol 2015;168(6):845–53.

49. Hernandez-Pampaloni M, Takalkar A, Yu JQ, et al. F-18 FDG-PET imaging and correlation with CT in staging and follow-up of pediatric lymphomas. Pediatr Radiol 2006;36(6):524–31.

50. Jadvar H, Connolly LP, Fahey FH, et al. PET and PET/CT in pediatric oncology. Semin Nucl Med 2007; 37(5):316–31.

51. Shammas A, Lim R, Charron M. Pediatric FDG PET/CT: physiologic uptake, normal variants, and benign conditions. Radiographics 2009;29(5):1467–86.

52. Barrington SF, O'Doherty MJ. Limitations of PET for imaging lymphoma. Eur J Nucl Med Mol Imaging 2003;30(Suppl 1):S117–27.

53. Bogot NR, Quint LE. Imaging of thymic disorders. Cancer Imaging 2005;5:139–49.

54. Kaste SC, Howard SC, McCarville EB, et al. 18F-FDG-avid sites mimicking active disease in pediatric Hodgkin's. Pediatr Radiol 2005;35(2):141–54.

55. Gawande RS, Khurana A, Messing S, et al. Differentiation of normal thymus from anterior mediastinal lymphoma and lymphoma recurrence at pediatric PET/CT. Radiology 2012;262(2):613–22.

56. Cheson BD, Fisher RI, Barrington SF, et al. Recommendations for initial evaluation, staging, and response assessment of Hodgkin and non-Hodgkin lymphoma: the Lugano classification. J Clin Oncol 2014;32(27):3059–68.

57. Barrington SF, Qian W, Somer EJ, et al. Concordance between four European centres of PET reporting criteria designed for use in multicentre trials in Hodgkin lymphoma. Eur J Nucl Med Mol Imaging 2010;37(10):1824–33.

58. Ahmed BA, Connolly BL, Shroff P, et al. Cumulative effective doses from radiologic procedures for pediatric oncology patients. Pediatrics 2010;126(4): e851–8.

59. Eissa HM, Allen CE, Kamdar K, et al. Pediatric Burkitt's lymphoma and diffuse B-cell lymphoma: are

surveillance scans required? Pediatr Hematol Oncol 2014;31(3):253–7.

60. DiMaggio C, Sun LS, Li G. Early childhood exposure to anesthesia and risk of developmental and behavioral disorders in a sibling birth cohort. Anesth Analg 2011;113(5):1143–51.

61. Stratmann G, Lee J, Sall JW, et al. Effect of general anesthesia in infancy on long-term recognition memory in humans and rats. Neuropsychopharmacology 2014;39(10):2275–87.

62. Atkin KL, Ditchfield MR. The role of whole-body MRI in pediatric oncology. J Pediatr Hematol Oncol 2014; 36(5):342–52.

63. Punwani S, Prakash V, Bainbridge A, et al. Quantitative diffusion weighted MRI: a functional biomarker of nodal disease in Hodgkin lymphoma? Cancer Biomark 2010;7(4):249–59.

64. Lin C, Luciani A, Itti E, et al. Whole-body diffusion-weighted magnetic resonance imaging with apparent diffusion coefficient mapping for staging patients with diffuse large B-cell lymphoma. Eur Radiol 2010;20(8):2027–38.

65. Littooij AS, Kwee TC, Barber I, et al. Whole-body MRI for initial staging of paediatric lymphoma:

prospective comparison to an FDG-PET/CT-based reference standard. Eur Radiol 2014;24(5):1153–65.

66. Siegel MJ, Jokerst CE, Rajderkar D, et al. Diffusion-weighted MRI for staging and evaluation of response in diffuse large B-cell lymphoma: a pilot study. NMR Biomed 2014;27(6):681–91.

67. Stephane V, Samuel B, Vincent D, et al. Comparison of PET-CT and magnetic resonance diffusion weighted imaging with body suppression (DWIBS) for initial staging of malignant lymphomas. Eur J Radiol 2013;82(11):2011–7.

68. Kwee TC, Takahara T, Ochiai R, et al. Diffusion-weighted whole-body imaging with background body signal suppression (DWIBS): features and potential applications in oncology. Eur Radiol 2008;18(9):1937–52.

69. Punwani S, Taylor SA, Saad ZZ, et al. Diffusion-weighted MRI of lymphoma: prognostic utility and implications for PET/MRI? Eur J Nucl Med Mol Imaging 2013;40(3):373–85.

70. Hirsch FW, Sattler B, Sorge I, et al. PET/MR in children. Initial clinical experience in paediatric oncology using an integrated PET/MR scanner. Pediatr Radiol 2013;43(7):860–75.

Imaging of Extranodal Genitourinary Lymphoma

 CrossMark

Iván R. Rohena-Quinquilla, MD[a,b], Grant E. Lattin Jr, MD[a,c], Darcy Wolfman, MD[a,c,d],*

KEYWORDS

- Lymphoma • Extranodal lymphoma • Genitourinary lymphoma • Primary extranodal lymphoma
- Lymphoma imaging • Lymphoma radiology • Lymphoma differential diagnosis

KEY POINTS

- Primary extranodal lymphoma in the genitourinary system is not as common as secondary involvement in disseminated lymphoma.
- A hypovascular, homogeneous mass arising from an organ in the genitourinary system with associated encasement of vessels should raise the suspicion of lymphoma, even in the absence of disseminated lymphoma.
- All primary extranodal GU lymphomas manifest around the age of 60 years, with the exception of primary gynecologic lymphoma which presents 1-2 decades earlier. Younger age at presentation is seen in immunocompromised patients which are at higher risk of developing lymphoma.
- While there are radiologic findings that can strongly suggest a prospective imaging diagnosis of primary extranodal GU lymphoma, it is critical to note that histologic confirmation is always necessary.

INTRODUCTION

The genitourinary (GU) system is commonly affected by disseminated lymphoma, also known as secondary extranodal disease. Rarely, lymphoma can originate from and remain localized to one of the GU organs and thus presents as primary extranodal disease. Although lymphoma more commonly manifests as nodal disease affecting lymph nodes and lymphoid organs (such as the spleen, thymus, tonsils, and pharyngeal lymphatic ring), up to 40% of lymphoma cases present as extranodal disease with only 3% having the GU system as the primary site of involvement.[1]

Non-Hodgkin lymphoma (NHL) constitutes most of the cases of GU lymphoma, with diffuse large B-cell lymphoma (DLBCL) as the predominant subtype.[2–5] Similar to other pathologic processes,

lymphoma has a limited pattern of cellular growth that can be classified as either expansile or infiltrative.[2,4,6–8] The predominant type of lymphomatous growth dictates some of the imaging features. Histologic attributes, such as cellular density, neovascularity, cystic degeneration/necrosis, and calcifications, can also be manifested on radiologic studies and provide additional imaging characteristics. These features result in multiple patterns, which, in addition to the potential for arising in virtually any tissue in the body, allows lymphoma to be described as one of the great imitators.

Despite its varied imaging appearance, a prospective imaging consideration for GU lymphoma is possible when certain characteristic imaging features are recognized (**Box 1**). This process is critical because, in contradistinction to the more common

Disclosure: The authors have nothing to disclose.
[a] Department of Radiology and Radiological Sciences, F. Edward Hébert School of Medicine, Uniformed Services University of the Health Sciences, 4301 Jones Bridge Road, Bethesda, MD 20814, USA; [b] Department of Radiology, Martin Army Community Hospital, 6600 Van Aalst Boulevard, Fort Benning, GA 31905-5637, USA; [c] American Institute for Radiologic Pathology, 1010 Wayne Avenue, Suite 320, Silver Spring, MD 20910, USA; [d] Department of Radiology, Walter Reed National Military Medical Center, 8901 Wisconsin Avenue, Bethesda, MD 20814, USA
* Corresponding author. 1010 Wayne Avenue, Suite 320, Silver Spring, MD 20910.
E-mail address: dwolfman@acr.org

Radiol Clin N Am 54 (2016) 747–764
http://dx.doi.org/10.1016/j.rcl.2016.03.009

radiologic.theclinics.com

Box 1
Diagnostic criteria for primary extranodal GU lymphoma

1. Lymphomatous disease confined to a GU organ.

2. If disease extends beyond the confines of a GU organ it should be limited to its immediate adjacent space, which may include nearby draining lymph nodes.

3. Simultaneous involvement of paired GU organs does not imply disseminated disease, provided (1) and (2) are met.

4. Disseminated disease arising from a primary GU site can be presumed when distant nodal disease is less extensive than at the GU site; however, this distinction usually does not affect treatment.

nonlymphomatous GU malignancies which is treated surgically, primary GU lymphoma is generally treated with chemotherapy and/or radiation therapy. Thus, by raising the possibility of GU lymphoma in the differential diagnosis, astute radiologists can offer percutaneous imaging-guided biopsy in an attempt to avoid unnecessary surgical intervention.

This review article describes and correlates the radiologic and pathologic features of extranodal lymphomatous disease affecting the GU system with specific focus on the kidneys, adrenal glands, testicles, and ovaries. Lymphomas of the uterine body and cervix, external female genitalia, urinary bladder, and prostate gland are briefly discussed (**Table 1**).

Renal Lymphoma

Primary renal lymphoma (PRL) is exceedingly rare; it accounts for less than 1% of all extranodal lymphomas.[1,9] In contrast, in the setting of disseminated lymphoma, the kidney is the most commonly involved GU organ, with up to 30% to 60% of cases detected in autopsy.[9–11] However, secondary involvement of the kidney by lymphoma is only detected in 3% to 8% of cases by imaging.[4,12] This wide discrepancy may be in part related to suboptimal detection of early renal disease by conventional anatomic imaging and lack of pathologic confirmation in the setting of renal involvement by disseminated disease.[2]

Clinical features

PRL is most commonly seen in middle-aged men.[13] Patients are usually asymptomatic and with unaffected renal function.[13] However, patients can present with flank pain, fatigue,

weight loss, hematuria, proteinuria, and renal failure.[14,15] Younger age at presentation can be seen in immunocompromised patients, who are at significantly higher risk for developing lymphoma.[16] The treatment of PRL and secondary renal lymphoma (SRL) is similar to its nodal counterpart, with the use of systemic chemotherapy.[17] Less commonly, nephrectomy or isolated radiation therapy have been described for the treatment of PRL.[18] Despite aggressive treatment, prognosis remains poor, with a 5-year survival rate of 29% for SRL and 40% to 50% for PRL.[17] Furthermore, the presence of renal involvement by disseminated lymphoma carries a high risk of central nervous system (CNS) relapse.[17]

Normal anatomy and imaging technique

The renal parenchyma is thought to contain no lymphoid tissue under normal circumstances, which explains the rarity of PRL.[2,4,9,13] Similar to other extranodal organs that lack lymphoid tissue, seeding of lymphoid cells from prior infection or inflammation is thought to play a role in the development of PRL.[1,9] In addition, the rich lymphatic networks that are normally present in the renal capsule and perirenal space can be a source of lymphoma, with subsequent spread to the renal parenchyma.[19,20] In SLR, the kidney can be involved by hematogenous spread or by capsular penetration caused by direct extension from preexisting perirenal space disease.[2,4]

Contrast-enhanced computed tomography (CT) is the imaging modality of choice for the detection, characterization, and staging of renal lymphoma.[4] Magnetic resonance (MR) imaging, with its better soft tissue contrast when compared with CT, has similar accuracy in the detection of renal lymphoma.[21] Because of its hypovascularity, renal lymphoma is best depicted in the nephrographic phase of imaging when both renal cortex and medulla are homogeneously opacified by contrast material.[9] Although the clinical utility of PET-CT for initial staging and monitoring of patients with lymphoma has been well established, newer techniques using whole-body diffusion-weighted (DW) MR imaging and PET-MR imaging are emerging.[22–24] Evaluation of renal lymphoma with ultrasonography (US) is limited because of its nonspecific imaging findings but can prove useful in patients with impaired renal function and for percutaneous imaging-guided renal biopsy.[25–27] With advancements in technique and diagnostic accuracy, the sensitivity and specificity for percutaneous imaging-guided renal biopsy in diagnosing malignancy reaches 90% to 100%.[28,29]

Table 1

Imaging and clinical features of primary extranodal GU lymphoma

GU Organ	Age (y)/Sex	% of All Primary Extranodal NHL	Symptoms	Treatment	5-y Survival Rate (%)	US	CT	MR Imaging
Kidney	60/Male	<1	Most asymptomatic; may present with flank pain, hematuria, and renal failure	Chemotherapy	40–50	Hypoechoic; may mimic a cyst	NonCon: slightly hyperdense; no fat or Ca^{2+} Con: homogeneously hypoenhancing	T1: hypointense; T2: isointense to hypointense Minimal homogeneous enhancement
Adrenal	62/Male	3	Highly symptomatic; B symptoms, abdominal pain, fatigue, and adrenal insufficiency	Chemotherapy	20 (1-y)	Hypoechoic, heterogenous	NonCon: hypodense; no fat or Ca^{2+} Con: slight to moderate enhancement	T1: hypointense T2: hyperintense Minimal or mild enhancement
Testicle	67	4	Painless testicular swelling; B symptoms uncommon	Orchiectomy + chemotherapy + radiation therapy	87	Hypoechoic, homogeneous Increased color flow vascularity	Nonspecific	T1 and T2 hypointense Prominent, heterogeneous enhancement
Ovarian	>40	<0.5	Abdominal/pelvic mass or pain; B symptoms; ascites	Oophorectomy (typical done for diagnosis) + chemotherapy	57	Bilateral, homogeneous, hypoechoic	Solid, large, homogeneous, hypovascular; ± solid peritoneal implants	T1: hypointense T2: intermediate to high SI Mild-moderate heterogeneous enhancement
Uterus/cervix	40–50	<1	Uterine or vaginal bleeding	Chemotherapy ± radiation therapy	67–100	Large, homogeneous mass or diffuse organ enlargement	Solid; mild-moderate enhancement	T1: hypointense T2: intermediate to high SI Hypovascular T2 zonal architecture preservation
Bladder	64/Female	<<0.5	Gross hematuria, urinary frequency, and dysuria	Radiation therapy ± chemotherapy	Good	Single, large, submucosal mass	Solitary mass (70%), single, large, multiple masses (20%), submucosal mass or diffuse wall thickening (10%)	Enhancing intravesical mass
Prostate	62	<<0.5	Bladder obstruction and renal failure; normal PSA	Variable, multimodality	33	Hypoechoic mass or masses	Homogeneous, solid mass or masses	Nonspecific

Abbreviations: Ca^{2+}, calcifications; Con, contrast material enhanced CT; NonCon, noncontrast material CT; MR, magnetic resonance; PSA, prostate-specific antigen test; SI, signal intensity; US, ultrasonography.

Imaging and pathologic findings

General PRL is manifested by lymphomatous disease limited to the kidney or immediate perirenal space. In contrast, SRL involves the presence of extensive extrarenal disease, typically with prominent retroperitoneal adenopathy. The imaging findings of PRL are similar to those in SRL with the exception of disseminated extrarenal disease present in the latter and absent in the former.[9] A definite diagnosis of PRL requires histologic confirmation and the exclusion of extrarenal disease at the time of diagnosis by bone marrow biopsy and initial staging whole-body imaging.[30]

The type of histologic growth pattern of lymphoma dictates some of its imaging features.[7] Radial growth is manifested on anatomic imaging as an expansile mass, which can be multiple (50%–60% of cases), involving 1 or both kidneys, or solitary (10%–25% of cases)[4] (**Box 2, Figs. 1** and **2**). The other type of lymphomatous growth pattern is infiltrative and can result in diffuse renal infiltration (20% of cases), direct capsular penetration from contiguous retroperitoneal disease (25%–30% of cases), or perirenal disease caused by direct extension from retroperitoneal disease or transcapsular spread of renal parenchymal disease[4,6] (**Box 3, Fig. 3**). An uncommon form of isolated perirenal disease is seen in less than 10% of cases and does not invade the renal parenchyma[4,31] (**Fig. 4**). To our knowledge, this unique

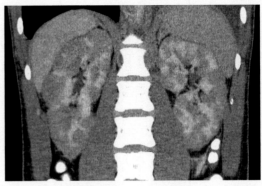

Fig. 1. Coronal postcontrast CT image showing multiple bilateral renal masses in a patient with secondary renal lymphoma.

form of renal lymphomatous disease has not been described in other GU organs.

Renal lymphomatous masses show variable size when radial growth predominates but are typically 1.0 to 4.5 cm in diameter.[4,8] Metastases, renal infarcts, septic emboli, and infection are all included in the imaging differential diagnosis when lymphoma presents as multiple renal masses, which is its most common pattern of renal involvement.[32] In such cases, the clinical history can be used to narrow the imaging considerations.

When renal infiltration predominates, the only anatomic abnormality may be renal enlargement with preservation of the reniform morphology[4,9] (see **Fig. 3**). Preferential involvement of the renal sinus and peripelvic region is an atypical pattern of lymphoma that usually results in minimal hydronephrosis for the degree of renal hilar encasement, and the renal vessels often remain patent[4,33] (**Fig. 5**). This pattern of renal lymphoma can be difficult to distinguish from Castleman disease of the renal sinus, but it is atypical for the more prevalent transitional cell carcinoma of the renal pelvis.[33,34] Complete renal encasement without parenchymal compression, destruction, or functional impairment infrequently occurs with perirenal lymphoma.[4] However, this finding is not pathognomonic for renal lymphoma because subcapsular hematoma, urinoma, retroperitoneal fibrosis, amyloidosis, extramedullary hematopoiesis, renal capsule sarcoma, perinephric space metastasis, immunoglobulin G4 sclerosing disease, and histiocytoses such as Erdheim-Chester disease demonstrate similar imaging appearance.[18,20] In agreement with these imaging findings, lymphomatous nodes and conglomerate masses are thus considered soft, in contrast with those from metastatic adenocarcinoma, which tend to be hard and result in hydronephrosis and renal vasculature invasion and obstruction.[8]

Box 2
Imaging differential diagnosis of renal lymphoma with expansile growth

Lymphoma: hypoenhancing; multiple masses or solitary; no calcifications; search for adjacent lymphadenopathy

Clear cell renal cell carcinoma (RCC): echogenic and heterogeneous composition and enhancement; vascular invasion; calcifications (11%)

Papillary and chromophobe RCC: hypoenhancing; well circumscribed; calcifications (up to 40% of cases)

Oncocytoma: well circumscribed; enhancement similar to renal cortex; may have a central scar; no adenopathy or vascular invasion

Angiomyolipoma: lobulated contour; heterogeneous enhancement; macroscopic fat (5% without identifiable fat); parenchymal defect with vessels traversing; pseudoaneurysms; hemorrhage when increased size

Metastasis: common primaries include lung, breast, colon, melanoma

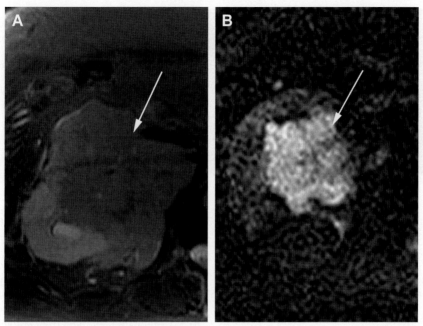

Fig. 2. Axial T2 fat saturation (*A*) and axial DW imaging (*B*) showing a renal hilar mass with hypointensity on T2 images (*arrow* in *A*) and restricted diffusion (*arrow* in *B*) in a patient with PRL.

Box 3
Imaging differential diagnosis of renal lymphoma with infiltrative growth

Neoplastic

Lymphoma: hypoenhancing; ill defined, may show increased renal size, pericapsular spread, or renal sinus involvement; search for adjacent lymphadenopathy

Urothelial carcinoma (transitional cell carcinoma [TCC]): hypoenhancing; may invade kidney; assess for component within the renal collecting system, vascular invasion, decreased or absent intravenous (IV) contrast material excretion

Renal medullary carcinoma: young age (<40 years); history of sickle cell trait; ill defined; renal enlargement; echogenic and heterogeneous composition

Renal collecting duct carcinoma: rare; hypoenhancing; central location with cortical extension; hyperechoic; T2 hypointense; mimics urothelial carcinoma

Squamous cell carcinoma: less common than TCC; originates in urothelium; may be preceded by chronic inflammation/infection (such as, xanthogranulomatous pyelonephritis [XGP]); aggressive growth; nonfunctional kidney; renal calculi are common

Metastasis: common primaries include lung, breast, colon, melanoma

Infectious/inflammatory

Pyelonephritis: hypoechoic or hyperechoic; striated nephrogram; may be focal; appropriate clinical setting

XGP: unilateral and diffuse; staghorn calculus (up to 70% of cases); hypodense centrally with thinned parenchyma mimicking hydronephrosis; decreased or absent IV contrast material excretion

Malakoplakia: rare; inflammatory mass with renal enlargement; variable echogenicity; ill defined, hypodense at CT; renal calculi are rare; bladder involvement more common than kidney

Tuberculosis: inflammatory mass; dystrophic calcifications; infundibular stenosis, amputated calyx, parenchymal scarring; low-density or calcified lymph nodes

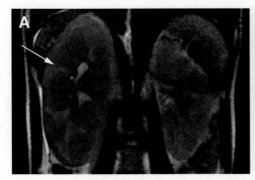
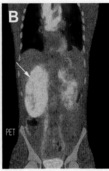

Fig. 3. Coronal T2 (*A*) and coronal PET (*B*) images showing diffuse renal enlargement of the right kidney (*arrows*) with corresponding marked fluorodeoxyglucose uptake on PET in a patient with PRL. Note that the right kidney maintains a normal reniform shape.

Following treatment of renal lymphoma most lymphomatous deposits disappear; however, cystic degeneration, necrosis, and calcifications may rarely develop[2] (see **Fig. 4**). In the absence of previous treatment, calcification in renal lymphoma is extremely rare.[35] Renal atrophy has also been documented following treatment of renal lymphoma.[2]

Pathology At histologic analysis, lymphoma is characterized by monotonous round blue cells with prominent round nuclei and scant cytoplasm.[4,6] These features render lymphoma a homogeneous process at imaging. For example, at US evaluation this homogeneity translates into minimal tissue interfaces with consequent low echogenicity.[4] In addition, the high cellularity and high nucleus/cytoplasm ratio in lymphoma results in a lower apparent diffusion coefficient value compared with other tumors. This histologic property is exploited by DW-MR imaging and results in restricted diffusion.

Atypical features of renal lymphoma include cystic degeneration, necrosis, and hemorrhage.[4] All of these histologic attributes result in loss of the usual homogeneous echogenicity, attenuation, and signal of lymphoma at US, CT, and MR imaging, respectively. Invasion and/or obstruction of the renal vasculature, hydronephrosis, and

calcifications are atypical manifestations that make other diagnoses more common than that of renal lymphoma.[8,13]

Despite increased stromal hemangiogenesis at histologic evaluation of aggressive lymphomas, the imaging findings of renal lymphoma are those of a hypovascular tumor with consequent minimal to no enhancement after the administration of intravenous (IV) contrast agents.[4,36] DLBCL is the most common histologic subtype in PRL.[1]

Ultrasonography The sonographic findings of renal lymphoma are nonspecific; however, most cases show hypoechogenicity in the lymphomatous deposits[9]; renal lymphoma can be mistaken for a simple renal cyst at sonographic evaluation.[4] Furthermore, when multiple renal lymphomatous deposits are present, it can resemble polycystic kidney disease.[2] In contrast, renal cell carcinoma (RCC) tends to be more echogenic than lymphoma at US.[4] Despite its diagnostic shortcomings, US has been proved useful for imaging-guided percutaneous biopsy, with core biopsies providing higher yield than fine-needle aspiration.[26,37]

Computed tomography Although renal lymphoma tends to be of slightly higher attenuation than the surrounding renal parenchyma, with an attenuation value of 30 to 50 Hounsfield units (HU) on unenhanced CT, it is characteristically of lower

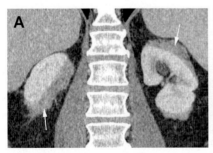
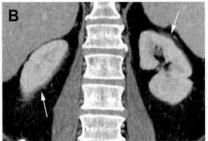

Fig. 4. Coronal postcontrast CT images before (*A*) and after (*B*) chemotherapy in a patient with PRL. Note the perirenal soft tissue before chemotherapy (*arrows* in *A*), which are resolved after chemotherapy (*arrows* in *B*).

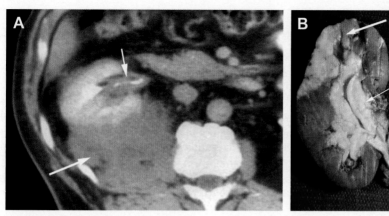

Fig. 5. Axial postcontrast CT image (*A*) showing perihilar (*white arrow* in *A*) and perirenal (*white bold arrow* in *A*) involvement in a patient with primary renal lymphoma. Note the lack of hydronephrosis. Corresponding gross photograph (*B*) showing the perihilar (*white arrow* in *B*) and perirenal (*white bold arrow* in *B*) involvement.

attenuation than the renal cortex on contrast-enhanced CT.[4,9,38] The hyperattenuating feature of renal lymphoma on unenhanced CT is an imaging consequence of the histologic property of hypercellularity in lymphomatous deposits. In the absence of cystic degeneration, renal lymphoma typically manifests as a homogeneous and hypovascular process affecting the renal parenchyma or perirenal space (see **Figs. 1**, **4**, and **5**). When involving the renal parenchyma, the imaging pattern may be indistinguishable from papillary and chromophobe RCC because both are often hypoattenuating on CT; however, it significantly differ from the heterogeneous attenuation and enhancement of the more prevalent clear cell RCC.[39,40]

Magnetic resonance imaging Renal lymphoma is commonly homogeneously hypointense on T1-weighted sequences with signal intensity lower than that of the normal renal cortex, isointense to hypointense on T2-weighted sequences, and shows minimal homogeneous enhancement that is less intense than the normal renal parenchyma after the administration of IV gadolinium-based contrast material[41] (see **Fig. 3**). Nonetheless, heterogeneous T2 signal hyperintensity and mild heterogeneous enhancement have also been reported.[21,41] In addition to its similar imaging features at CT, papillary RCC is also characteristically hypointense on T2-weighted sequences, making imaging differentiation from PRL with expansile growth difficult.[42] With the use of whole-body DW-MR imaging it is possible to identify renal involvement by lymphoma.[24]

PET/computed tomography Because of its increased metabolic activity, most lymphomas have high-grade fluorodeoxyglucose (FDG) uptake

and are therefore well depicted by PET/CT imaging (see **Fig. 3**). Renal lymphomas often show intense FDG avidity comparable with the adjacent normal renal parenchyma, which differs from the low-level FDG uptake of RCC.[9] However, there is no specific standardized uptake value ratio that indicates renal disorder and physiologic FDG excretion by normally functioning kidneys also limits the sensitivity of PET imaging for detecting renal neoplasms.[43]

Adrenal Lymphoma

Primary adrenal lymphoma (PAL) is an extremely rare entity with approximately 200 cases reported in the English literature.[44,45] As such, it accounts for less than 1% of all NHLs and 3% of primary extranodal lymphomas.[1,44] Similar to SRL, adrenal gland involvement by disseminated lymphomatous disease is seen in up to 25% of autopsy series but only in 4% of cases by CT imaging.[46–48] PAL should only be diagnosed if there is biopsy-proven lymphoma involving 1 or both adrenal glands in the absence of prior history or evidence of lymphoma elsewhere.[45] If abnormal lymph nodes are present, the disease should be limited to the space adjacent to the adrenal glands (**Box 4**).

Clinical features
PAL is an aggressive disease that predominately affects elderly men, with a mean age at presentation of 62 years and a male/female ratio of approximately 1.8:1.[45] It results in highly symptomatic disease with 68% of cases presenting with B symptoms, followed by abdominal pain and fatigue in 42% and 36% of cases, respectively.[45] This presentation differs from secondary involvement of the adrenal glands by diffuse

---

Box 4
Imaging differential diagnosis of adrenal lymphoma

Lymphoma: PAL extremely rare; secondary adrenal lymphoma common; highly symptomatic; bilateral (up to 75%); typically hypovascular and large (8 cm); heterogeneous, hypoechoic; no calcifications; search for lymphadenopathy

Adrenal cortical adenoma: common; typically hypodense (<10 HU noncontrast density or >60% absolute washout); degenerating adenoma may have increased size, heterogeneity, hemorrhage, or calcification

Adrenal cortical carcinoma: younger age; often symptomatic; unilateral (90%); large (12 cm), heterogeneous composition and enhancement, and calcifications (30%); locally invasive, aggressive imaging features

Pheochromocytoma: classically increased urine metanephrine levels; may not be functional; metaiodobenzylguanidine avid; heterogeneous enhancement; typically T2 hyperintense; imaging may vary with low density, avid washout, and cystic component

Myelolipoma: contains macroscopic fat (typically >50%); well-circumscribed mass; may be bilateral; calcifications (24%)

Metastasis: common primaries include lung, breast, renal, and melanoma

---

lymphomatous disease in which most cases are clinically silent.[2] In most cases (50%–75%) of PAL there is bilateral adrenal gland involvement[45,49] (**Fig. 6**). This condition is strongly associated with adrenal insufficiency, which is seen in about 60% of cases of PAL.[45] Treatment is usually with chemotherapy, similar to other NHL. However, despite aggressive chemotherapy, the prognosis of PAL is dismal, with a 1-year survival rate of 20%.[45] Furthermore, the addition of adrenalectomy before chemotherapy is not associated with a survival benefit.[45]

Normal anatomy and imaging technique
The adrenals are paired endocrine glands that are usually considered part of the GU system given their location in the suprarenal space. Although there are no lymphatic vessels in the adrenal parenchyma, extensive subserous lymphatic

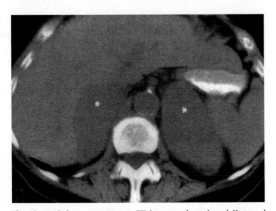

Fig. 6. Axial noncontrast CT image showing bilateral adrenal masses (*asterisks*) that proved to be PAL. Note the masses are hypodense at noncontrast CT.

networks overlie the adrenal gland and communicate with adrenal capsule lymphatics.[50] Lymphatic drainage is primarily toward the midline into the thoracic duct via a direct pathway or by way of regional lymph nodes.[50]

CT and MR imaging are the most commonly used modalities for characterization of adrenal lesions. With the use of an attenuation value less than 10 HU or an absolute washout of 60% or higher, CT imaging can effectively exclude adrenal malignancy to include adrenal lymphoma.[51] MR imaging can also be used to exclude adrenal lymphoma by showing macroscopic fat or intracellular lipid in an adrenal lesion.[49] Both PET/CT and whole-body DW imaging have been used for the detection of adrenal lymphoma.[24,52]

Imaging and pathologic findings
General and pathology As in other GU organs, adrenal lymphoma can manifest as a focal, multifocal, or infiltrative process. The most common presentation of PAL is as a large lymphomatous mass (median size of 8 cm) that replaces the normal adrenal gland morphology and is bilateral in up to 75% of cases[45] (see **Fig. 6**; **Fig. 7**). Despite having variable imaging characteristics, PAL should be considered in the setting of large, bilateral adrenal masses with mild to moderate enhancement that are hypodense on CT imaging, FDG-avid on PET/CT, and show low T1 signal and high T2 signal on MR imaging as well as restricted diffusion.[45] In secondary adrenal lymphoma, the glands may show normal size and morphology, diffuse enlargement while maintaining their normal shape, or have 1 or more masses.[53] Large tumors commonly infiltrate

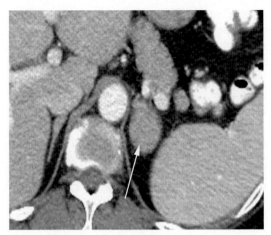

Fig. 7. Axial postcontrast CT image reveals a solitary adrenal mass (*arrow*) shown to be PAL.

adjacent structures.[54] Most cases of adrenal lymphoma are classified histologically as DLBCL.[44]

Ultrasonography The sonographic findings of adrenal lymphoma are nonspecific; however, most cases are heterogeneously hypoechoic.[45] A recent review of 11 cases of PAL showed that none of the cases was reported as homogeneously hyperechoic.[45] The heterogeneous echogenicity may be explained by the variable presence of hemorrhage or necrosis in these large masses.[45]

Computed tomography The CT appearance cannot be used as a discriminating factor because both homogeneous and heterogeneous attenuation are equally prevalent in PAL; however, hypodense masses are reported as being more common than hyperdense masses[45] (see **Fig. 6**). Of the 23 cases of PAL evaluated in a recent review, 18 cases were considered to show slight to moderate enhancement, whereas the rest showed no or limited enhancement.[45] In the absence of prior treatment, calcifications are exceeding rare in adrenal lymphoma.[55] Aggressive features, such as vascular invasion, as well as the presence of calcifications, strongly suggest the more prevalent adrenal cortical carcinoma as opposed to adrenal lymphoma.

Magnetic resonance imaging At MR imaging, adrenal lymphoma is typically manifested as low signal intensity on T1-weighted images, high signal intensity on T2-weighted images, and high signal on DW-MR imaging with restricted diffusion; minimal or mild progressive enhancement; and similar distribution of homogeneous and heterogeneous signal intensity.[45,49] The MR imaging appearance of adrenal lymphoma is similar to that of adrenal metastases, which are the most

common malignant lesions affecting the adrenal glands. Imaging-guided biopsy is a useful tool in the evaluation of adrenal lesions with equivocal imaging characteristics.[56]

PET/computed tomography Lymphomatous involvement of the adrenal glands tends to show a high degree of uptake on FDG-PET/CT which is of great utility to assess subtle disease that render the adrenals morphologically normal.[52] As such, it is imperative to note that preservation of the adreniform shape of 1 or both adrenal glands does not exclude adrenal disease.[52]

Testicular Lymphoma

Primary testicular lymphoma (PTL) is an uncommon malignancy that constitutes around 3% to 9% of all testicular cancers, 4% of extranodal NHL, and 1% to 2% of all NHL.[13,57,58] It is nonetheless the most common testicular neoplasm in men more than 60 years of age, accounting for 50% of cases in this age group.[58,59] This incidence contrasts with the more common primary testicular neoplasms, which affect young men and are classified histologically as germ cell tumors (GCTs) in 95% of cases.[60] Similar to other GU organs, secondary testicular lymphoma (STL) is more common than PTL[61] (**Box 5**).

Clinical features

Patients with PTL have a median age at presentation of 67 years, which significantly differs from GCT, which typically presents at 15 to 35 years of age.[58,60] Painless testicular swelling/enlargement is the most common clinical symptom for both PTL and GCT.[57,61] B symptoms are uncommon in PTL but, when present, are typically in the setting of advanced disease.[58,61] The most

---

Box 5
Imaging differential diagnosis of testicular lymphoma

Lymphoma: older men (>60 years); bilateral (up to 33%); homogeneously hypoechoic masses; increased Doppler color flow

GCTs: younger age (15–35 years); typically unilateral and homogeneously hypoechoic (seminoma) or heterogeneous (nonseminomatous GCTs)

Orchitis: clinical signs of infection; search for epididymal involvement; may be indistinguishable by imaging

Tuberculosis and sarcoidosis: may be indistinguishable by imaging; search for extratesticular imaging findings

frequent histology in PTL is DLBCL, accounting for 70% to 90% of cases.[57,58] Earlier presentation with a median age of 36 years is seen in human immunodeficiency virus–positive patients with PTL, albeit with different histologic subtypes (such as, immunoblastic, plasmablastic, or Burkitt-like lymphoma).[62]

Inguinal orchiectomy is the first-line therapeutic procedure of choice for PTL because it provides for both definite diagnosis and removal of a potential sanctuary site for lymphoma cells.[58,63] Irradiation of the contralateral testicle, CNS prophylaxis with intrathecal chemotherapy, and systemic chemotherapy are commonly used in the treatment plan.[58] With this multimodal therapeutic approach, the prognosis of PTL has significantly improved, with a 5-year overall survival of 87% for patients treated after 2000 compared with 56% for those treated between 1977 and 1999.[64]

Normal anatomy and imaging technique

The blood-testis barrier renders the testicles as immunoprivileged sites whereby chemotherapeutic agents may have reduced efficacy and lymphoma cells may escape the host T-cell antitumor response.[58] Note that although the scrotal lymphatic drainage is to the inguinal nodes, the testicles drain to the para-aortic and paracaval lymph nodes with occasional drainage to the ipsilateral pelvic nodes.[58,60] This drainage pathway is consistent with the embryologic origin of the testes and must be subject to close inspection by the radiologist.[58]

The testicles have been shown to contain parenchymal lymphatics located in the septula testis that connect with lymph vessels in the rete testis and tunica albuginea, which in turn drain into the spermatic cord lymphatics.[65]

US is the first-line imaging technique used in the evaluation of the testes given its high sensitivity (92%–98%) and specificity (95%–99.8%) for the evaluation of testicular malignancy.[60] Color Doppler US, in addition to gray-scale US, increases the conspicuity of round cell infiltration of the testicle by lymphoma.[66] The main goal of US testicular evaluation is to allow differentiation of intratesticular lesions, which are most commonly malignant, from extratesticular lesions, which are typically benign. CT imaging, with or without the use of PET/CT, is generally not used for the primary evaluation of testicular disease; however, it is of great value for initial staging and follow-up of patients with testicular malignancy, including lymphoma. Testicular MR imaging is usually not required to guide patient management when US shows an intratesticular mass and, as such, is most commonly used as a problem-solving diagnostic modality.[67] A high sensitivity and specificity (100% and 88%, respectively) for differentiating benign from malignant intratesticular disease has been shown with MR imaging.[68]

Imaging and pathologic findings

General PTL is defined as lymphomatous disease limited to 1 or both testicles with or without the presence of limited extranodal disease at the time of diagnosis.[3,62] As previously discussed, disseminated disease has to be excluded in order to establish a definite diagnosis of primary extranodal lymphoma. The only way of differentiating PTL from STL on imaging is by careful evaluation of the extrascrotal contents, usually with CT or PET/CT.

At imaging, PTL is commonly seen as unilateral testicular enlargement with predilection for the right testicle given by a right/left testicular ratio of 1.6:1.[57,61,63,69] Nonetheless, there is considerable variation in the rate of bilateral involvement at imaging, ranging from 0% in one recent series of 9 patients with PTL to 33% in a series of 12 patients.[57,63] The lymphomatous deposits vary in size from 0.8 cm to greater than 5 cm with extratesticular extension.[66,70]

Pathology The histologic changes of a diffusely infiltrating testicular process without destruction are well translated into imaging. With a monotonous atypical cellular arrangement surrounding and compressing the seminiferous tubules and uncommon presence of tumoral hemorrhage and necrosis, testicular lymphoma is seen at imaging as a focal, multifocal, or infiltrative homogeneous process with preservation of the normal ovoid testicular shape.[2] These histologic characteristics differ from those of nonseminomatous GCTs (NSGCT) in which blood vessel invasion, which commonly leads to necrosis and hemorrhage, results in heterogeneous echogenicity and heterogeneous T2 signal hyperintensity at US and MR imaging, respectively.[71]

A distinctive feature of testicular lymphoma is its tendency to spread to the epididymis and spermatic cord, which is less commonly seen with GCT.[2,70,72] Up to 90% of PTLs are diffuse large B-cell type and, as such, express typical B-cell markers: CD19, CD20, CD79a, and PAX5.[58,62]

Ultrasonography Testicular lymphoma is characteristically homogeneously hypoechoic with increased color flow vascularity irrespective of tumor size[61,66,69] (**Fig. 8**). The reason behind the increased Doppler color flow is not completely understood and the flow is dissimilar to lymphoma elsewhere in the GU system. Small testicular hydroceles can also be seen.[66,69] At US, the imaging

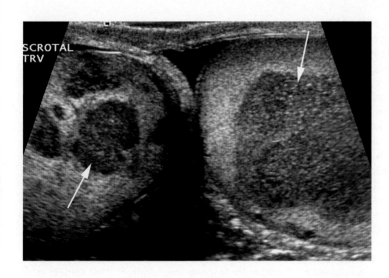

Fig. 8. Transverse gray-scale ultrasonography image through both testicles showing bilateral hypoechoic masses (*arrows*) in a patient with PTL.

findings of testicular lymphoma can be indistinguishable from those of epididymo-orchitis, tuberculosis, sarcoidosis, leukemia, and seminoma. However, in addition to clinical symptoms and laboratory evaluation, older age at presentation favors lymphoma rather than infection and seminoma.

MR imaging Compared with the normal testicular parenchyma, testicular lymphoma tends to be hypointense in both T1-weighted and T2-weighted MR images.[73] This signal intensity combination pattern has been associated with testicular malignancy, including seminoma.[68,72] After the administration of IV gadolinium, PTL has shown strong and heterogeneous enhancement.[74]

PET/computed tomography PET/CT has been shown to be more sensitive than CT alone for assessing lymphomatous disease at initial staging as well as in follow-up evaluation.[22] However, when the disease is confined to the testicular parenchyma, such as in PTL, it might be impossible to distinguish pathologic lymphoma cell FDG uptake from normal physiologic testicular activity.[22]

Female Genital Tract Lymphoma

Primary extranodal gynecologic lymphoma is exceedingly rare with an estimated 165 cases occurring annually in the United States.[75] This incidence is in contradistinction with the approximate 1650 to 2500 cases per year of secondary involvement of the gynecologic tract by disseminated lymphoma.[75] The ovary is the most common gynecologic organ involved in both primary and secondary extranodal lymphoma.[75] After the ovaries, the uterine cervix, uterine corpus, and vagina

follow in decreasing order of frequency.[75] Primary vulvar and fallopian tube lymphomas are extraordinarily rare.[75]

Ovarian lymphoma

Primary ovarian lymphoma (POL) is a rare malignancy that accounts for 1.5% of all ovarian neoplasms and only 0.14% to 0.5% of all cases of extranodal lymphoma.[5,76,77] In contrast, up to 26% of cases of disseminated lymphoma involve the ovary at autopsy.[77] The most common histologic type is DLBCL, followed by Burkitt lymphoma, which accounts for 50% of pediatric ovarian malignancies.[5]

Clinical features The age at presentation for POL has a wide range but is most commonly seen in women more than 40 years of age.[78] Although abdominopelvic pain or mass is the most common presentation, ascites and B symptoms can also be present.[79] Similar to primary ovarian malignancies, the blood serum marker CA-125 is frequently increased.[80,81] Treatment is most commonly in the form of systemic chemotherapy; however, initial oophorectomy is frequently performed as a means of histologic diagnosis.[5,80] The prognosis of POL is poor despite aggressive chemotherapy, with a 5-year survival rate of 57%.[82]

Normal anatomy and imaging technique Lymphocytes are present in the vessels of the ovarian hilum and within the corpus luteum.[5,83] However, contrary to popular belief, the normal ovarian parenchyma does contain sporadic parenchymal lymphocytes of both T-cell and B-cell lineage.[77,79,84] These cells might be involved in the lymphogenesis of POL.

The 3 main routes of ovarian lymphatic drainage are from the ovarian veins to the para-aortic and paracaval lymph nodes; from the broad ligament to the internal and external iliac lymph nodes and to the junctional nodes at the junction between the internal and external iliac nodal groups; and from the round ligament to the inguinal lymph nodes.[85]

US remains by far the most commonly used imaging modality to assess ovarian disease. Differentiating benign disease from malignancy is often possible when certain sonographic features are present.[86] CT imaging is not usually used for the primary evaluation of ovarian disorders; however, with the increased routine use of CT, many ovarian masses are first detected with this imaging modality. MR imaging provides the best imaging characterization of ovarian masses and has been shown to significantly alter clinical management in patients with indeterminate pelvic findings on US or CT.[87] Although there are currently no data to confirm the appropriateness of PET/CT in POL, it is presumed to be of clinical utility given its central role in the imaging of other lymphomas.

Imaging and pathologic findings Similar to other GU organs, POL should be diagnosed when the lymphomatous deposits are confined to the ovary, regional lymph nodes, or adjacent organs at the time of initial diagnosis; bone marrow and peripheral blood do not contain abnormal cells; and, if extraovarian disease appears later, there must be a few months between the time ovarian and extraovarian lesions are detected.[88]

Ovarian lymphomas are commonly displayed as large, bilateral, solid ovarian masses at imaging. Tumor size is a critical feature because almost all masses are greater than 5 cm, with a mean diameter of 10 to 15 cm.[77,79] Ascites is an inconsistent finding.[79,89]

The histologic changes of ovarian lymphoma resemble those of lymphoma elsewhere in the GU tract with diffuse malignant lymphoid cells infiltrating, but not destroying, the ovarian parenchyma and occasional areas of cystic degeneration and necrosis that alter the typical homogeneous architecture at imaging. Fallopian tube involvement is common.[5]

The US findings of ovarian lymphoma are nonspecific but are most commonly manifested as homogeneously hypoechoic masses with minimal color Doppler vascularity.[89] This finding is in contradistinction with the more common tumors of the ovarian surface epithelium (serous and mucinous tumors), which are predominantly cystic. However, heterogeneous echogenicity with solid and cystic components has also been described in POL.[90] Similarly, CT typically shows solid, homogeneous, and hypovascular ovarian masses.[89] At MR imaging, ovarian lymphoma is characteristically hypointense on T1-weighted images, intermediate to high signal intensity on T2-weighted images, and minimal to moderate heterogeneously enhancing after the administration of IV gadolinium-based contrast agents[91] (**Fig. 9**). Ovarian fibromas/fibrothecomas and Brenner tumors are solid ovarian masses that

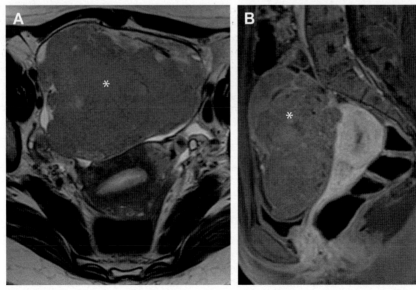

Fig. 9. Axial T2 (*A*) and coronal T1 post–fat saturation (*B*) images showing an intermediate T2 signal mass (*asterisk* in *A*) with minimal enhancement postcontrast (*asterisk* in *B*) in a patient with POL.

can be distinguished from POL by their smaller size, predominant unilaterality, and dramatic T2 signal hypointensity, which results from the high fibrous content in these tumors.[92] Peripherally placed ovarian follicles, such as in ovarian torsion and granulocytic sarcoma (chloroma), have also been described in ovarian lymphoma[93,94] (**Box 6**).

Uterine body and cervical lymphoma

Primary uterine lymphoma is uncommon. It represents less than 1% of all extranodal lymphomas and is much more common in the uterine cervix than it is in the uterine body.[5] Patients most commonly present with abnormal uterine or vaginal bleeding at the age of 40 to 50 years.[95,96] The most common histologic subtype for both uterine body and cervical lymphoma is DLBCL.[96] Secondary uterine lymphoma in the setting of advanced lymphomatous disease is far more common than the primary form.[13] Treatment is typically with systemic chemotherapy with or without the use of radiation therapy. The prognosis for primary uterine lymphoma is good, with a 5-year survival rate of 67% to 100%.[97]

The imaging findings of cervical lymphoma are nonspecific and frequently show a large uterine mass or diffuse uterine enlargement with or without adjacent organ spread.[5] The MR imaging findings of cervical lymphoma are variable and usually indistinguishable from those of cervical carcinoma. Lymphomatous involvement of the cervix tends to be homogeneously hypointense on T1-weighted images, intermediate to high homogeneous signal intensity on T2-weighted images, and hypovascular with preservation of the T2 zonal architecture at MR imaging.[98–100]

Uterine body lymphoma has a similar imaging appearance to cervical lymphoma and is characterized by a large homogeneous mass with mild to moderate uniform enhancement.[5] Preservation of the zonal anatomy may or may not be present.[5,101]

Vaginal and vulvar lymphoma

Lymphoma of the vagina and vulva is extremely rare. Presentation is in the 40s for vaginal lymphoma and late 50s for vulvar lymphoma.[5] DLBCL is the most common type of lymphoma affecting both of these sites.[5] The imaging findings of vaginal lymphoma are similar to those of uterine lymphoma.[5] There are no reports on the imaging finding of primary vulvar lymphoma.

Urinary Bladder Lymphoma

Primary bladder lymphoma (PBL) is exceeding rare, with fewer than 100 cases reported to date.[102] Secondary involvement of the urinary bladder by disseminated lymphomatous disease is more common than primary disease and occurs in 10% to 25% of cases.[102] The mean age at presentation is 64 years and the female/male ratio is 3:1,[102] which contrasts with the male predominance of primary urinary bladder cancer.[103] There is a statistically significant predilection for Caucasians.[13] A clinical triad of gross hematuria, urinary frequency, and dysuria are commonly encountered, as is a history of chronic cystitis.[102] On histology, most cases are low-grade non-Hodgkin B-cell lymphomas of mucosa-associated lymphoid tissue (MALT) subtype.[102] The treatment of PBL is most commonly with radiation therapy and the prognosis is good.[102]

Bladder lymphoma is most frequently seen at imaging as a solitary mass in 70% of cases and, less commonly, as multiple masses or diffuse

---

Box 6
Imaging differential diagnosis of ovarian lymphoma

Lymphoma: older age (>40 years); large (10–15 cm), bilateral, solid, and homogeneous; intermediate to high signal intensity on T2-weighted images; no calcifications

Serous and mucinous ovarian tumors (epithelial surface tumor): wide age range (typically >20 years); predominantly cystic masses; typically unilateral in mucinous and bilateral in serous; peritoneal spread

Fibrothecoma (sex cord–stroma tumor): older age (>40 years); unilateral, large (13 cm), and very hypovascular; very low T2 signal intensity

Dysgerminoma (germ cell tumor): younger age (most <20 years); unilateral (90%–95%), large (15 cm), and hypervascular; multilobulated solid mass divided by fibrovascular septae; lymphatic spread

Brenner tumor (epithelial-stromal tumor): 30 to 70 years of age; small (<5 cm), unilateral (>85%); completely solid or with cystic elements; very low T2 signal intensity with mild to moderate enhancement; calcifications; associated with other epithelial neoplasms in same ovary (up to 20%)

Metastasis: common primaries include gastrointestinal tract, endometrium, breast, and skin; particularly in premenopausal age

bladder wall thickening.[102] It usually involves the submucosa without mucosal ulceration.[2] The radiologic findings are nonspecific and cannot be differentiated from other bladder neoplasms by imaging alone.[104]

Prostate Lymphoma

Primary prostate lymphoma (PPL) is extremely rare, with fewer than 100 cases reported. It constitutes 0.1% of all NHLs and 0.1% of all prostatic tumors.[13,105] Secondary involvement of the prostate gland by disseminated disease is more common than PPL.[106] The mean age of presentation is 62 years.[106] Bladder outlet obstruction caused by prostatism, which often causes renal failure, is the most common presenting symptom.[106] Even though the imaging findings of prostatic lymphoma are nonspecific, cross-sectional imaging can be useful for staging.[107] The prognosis of prostate lymphoma, primary and secondary, is poor, with a 5-year survival rate of 33%.[106]

Pearls, pitfalls, variants

1. Most primary extranodal GU lymphomas manifest as a solid mass or masses of homogeneous composition. With the exception of PTL, GU lymphomas are hypovascular.
2. Heterogeneous echogenicity, attenuation, and signal can sometimes be seen at US, CT, and MR imaging, respectively, when there is cystic degeneration and necrosis; however, calcifications are extremely rare in GU lymphomas in the absence of prior treatment.
3. Because lymphoma tends to surround and encase structures, the presence of displacement and invasion of adjacent organs or vessels should make other diagnoses more common than that of lymphoma.
4. Isolated perirenal lymphoma, which mimics other neoplastic and nonneoplastic entities, is a unique form of GU lymphomatous disease that has not been described in other GU organs.
5. Renal lymphoma may mimic a renal cyst at US and can be indistinguishable from papillary and chromophobe RCC at CT and MR imaging when the RCCs do not contain calcifications.
6. Primary testicular and renal lymphomas may be difficult to identify on PET/CT because of the presence of normally increased FDG metabolic activity and excretion in these organs, respectively.

What referring physicians need to know

1. All primary extranodal GU lymphomas manifest around the age of 60 years, with the exception of primary gynecologic lymphoma, which presents 1 to 2 decades earlier. Younger age at presentation is seen in immunocompromised patients, who are at higher risk of developing lymphoma.
2. Although there are radiologic findings that can strongly suggest a prospective imaging diagnosis of primary extranodal GU lymphoma, it is critical to note that histologic confirmation is always necessary.
3. The most common histologic subtype in all primary extranodal GU lymphomas is DLBCL; however, MALT lymphoma is most common in PBL.
4. The treatment of primary extranodal GU lymphomas is primarily nonsurgical, with the exception of PTL, which requires orchiectomy as a diagnostic and therapeutic procedure.
5. Primary lymphomas of the testicle, bladder, and uterus have much better prognoses than the remainder of primary GU lymphomas.
6. The main differentiation between primary and secondary extranodal lymphomas of the GU system relies on proper initial staging with whole-body imaging (PET/CT and/or whole-body MR imaging) and bone marrow biopsy.
7. Differentiating between primary extranodal GU lymphoma with distant metastases and nodal lymphoma with GU metastases is often impossible, but is usually not necessary because the treatment is identical.

SUMMARY

Primary extranodal lymphoma can involve any GU organ independent of the existence of normally occurring parenchymal lymphoid cells in the index organ. The ability to recognize the varied imaging patterns of primary GU lymphoma enables radiologists to suggest a prospective diagnosis and engage in percutaneous imaging-guided biopsy as a means of establishing a histologic diagnosis in lieu of primary surgical intervention. This ability is expected to result in expedited treatment and decreased patient morbidity and mortality from avoidance of unnecessary surgery. Further, radiologists continue to engage in patient care during initial imaging, staging and follow-up monitoring of GU lymphomatous disease.

REFERENCES

1. Freeman C, Berg JW, Cutler SJ. Occurrence and prognosis of extranodal lymphomas. Cancer 1972;29(1):252–60.
2. Charnsangavej C. Lymphoma of the genitourinary tract. Radiol Clin North Am 1990;28(4):865–77.

3. Chua SC, Rozalli FI, O'Connor SR. Imaging features of primary extranodal lymphomas. Clin Radiol 2009;64(6):574–88.

4. Sheth S, Ali S, Fishman E. Imaging of renal lymphoma: patterns of disease with pathologic correlation. Radiographics 2006;26(4):1151–68.

5. Onyiuke I, Kirby AB, McCarthy S. Primary gynecologic lymphoma: imaging findings. AJR Am J Roentgenol 2013;201(4):W648–55.

6. Pickhardt PJ, Lonergan GJ, Davis CJ Jr, et al. From the archives of the AFIP. Infiltrative renal lesions: radiologic-pathologic correlation. Armed Forces Institute of Pathology. Radiographics 2000;20(1): 215–43.

7. Hartman DS, David CJ Jr, Goldman SM, et al. Renal lymphoma: radiologic-pathologic correlation of 21 cases. Radiology 1982;144(4):759–66.

8. Urban BA, Fishman EK. Renal lymphoma: CT patterns with emphasis on helical CT. Radiographics 2000;20(1):197–212.

9. Ganeshan D, Iyer R, Devine C, et al. Imaging of primary and secondary renal lymphoma. AJR Am J Roentgenol 2013;201(5):W712–9.

10. Kandel LB, McCullough DL, Harrison LH, et al. Primary renal lymphoma. Does it exist? Cancer 1987; 60(3):386–91.

11. Miyake O, Namiki M, Sonoda T, et al. Secondary involvement of genitourinary organs in malignant lymphoma. Urol Int 1987;42(5):360–2.

12. Bach AG, Behrmann C, Holzhausen HJ, et al. Prevalence and patterns of renal involvement in imaging of malignant lymphoproliferative diseases. Acta Radiol 2012;53(3):343–8.

13. Taheri MR, Dighe MK, Kolokythas O, et al. Multifaceted genitourinary lymphoma. Curr Probl Diagn Radiol 2008;37(2):80–93.

14. Kose F, Sakalli H, Mertsoylu H, et al. Primary renal lymphoma: report of four cases. Onkologie 2009; 32(4):200–2.

15. Hart S, Ellimoottil C, Shafer D, et al. A case of primary renal lymphoma. Urology 2012;80(4): 763–5.

16. Gibson TM, Engels EA, Clarke CA, et al. Risk of diffuse large B-cell lymphoma after solid organ transplantation in the United States. Am J Hematol 2014;89(7):714–20.

17. Villa D, Connors JM, Sehn LH, et al. Diffuse large B-cell lymphoma with involvement of the kidney: outcome and risk of central nervous system relapse. Haematologica 2011;96(7):1002–7.

18. Dedekam E, Graham J, Strenge K, et al. Primary renal lymphoma mimicking a subcapsular hematoma: a case report. J Radiol Case Rep 2013; 7(8):18–26.

19. Salem Y, Pagliaro LC, Manyak MJ. Primary small noncleaved cell lymphoma of kidney. Urology 1993;42(3):331–5.

20. Bechtold RE, Dyer RB, Zagoria RJ, et al. The perirenal space: relationship of pathologic processes to normal retroperitoneal anatomy. Radiographics 1996;16(4):841–54.

21. Hauser M, Krestin GP, Hagspiel KD. Bilateral solid multifocal intrarenal and perirenal lesions: differentiation with ultrasonography, computed tomography and magnetic resonance imaging. Clin Radiol 1995;50(5):288–94.

22. Cronin CG, Swords R, Truong MT, et al. Clinical utility of PET/CT in lymphoma. AJR Am J Roentgenol 2010;194(1):W91–103.

23. Gu J, Chan T, Zhang J, et al. Whole-body diffusion-weighted imaging: the added value to whole-body MRI at initial diagnosis of lymphoma. AJR Am J Roentgenol 2011;197(3):W384–91.

24. Toledano-Massiah S, Luciani A, Itti E, et al. Whole-body diffusion-weighted imaging in Hodgkin lymphoma and diffuse large B-cell lymphoma. Radiographics 2015;35(3):747–64.

25. Hesselmann V, Zahringer M, Krug B, et al. Computed-tomography-guided percutaneous core needle biopsies of suspected malignant lymphomas: impact of biopsy, lesion, and patient parameters on diagnostic yield. Acta Radiol 2004; 45(6):641–5.

26. Balestreri L, Morassut S, Bernardi D, et al. Efficacy of CT-guided percutaneous needle biopsy in the diagnosis of malignant lymphoma at first presentation. Clin Imaging 2005;29(2):123–7.

27. Beland MD, Mayo-Smith WW, Dupuy DE, et al. Diagnostic yield of 58 consecutive imaging-guided biopsies of solid renal masses: should we biopsy all that are indeterminate? AJR Am J Roentgenol 2007;188(3):792–7.

28. Maturen KE, Nghiem HV, Caoili EM, et al. Renal mass core biopsy: accuracy and impact on clinical management. AJR Am J Roentgenol 2007;188(2): 563–70.

29. Wang R, Wolf JS Jr, Wood DP Jr, et al. Accuracy of percutaneous core biopsy in management of small renal masses. Urology 2009;73(3):586–90 [discussion: 590–1].

30. Stallone G, Infante B, Manno C, et al. Primary renal lymphoma does exist: case report and review of the literature. J Nephrol 2000;13(5):367–72.

31. Leite NP, Kased N, Hanna RF, et al. Cross-sectional imaging of extranodal involvement in abdominopelvic lymphoproliferative malignancies. Radiographics 2007;27(6):1613–34.

32. Sheeran SR, Sussman SK. Renal lymphoma: spectrum of CT findings and potential mimics. AJR Am J Roentgenol 1998;171(4):1067–72.

33. Lee WK, Lau EW, Duddalwar VA, et al. Abdominal manifestations of extranodal lymphoma: spectrum of imaging findings. AJR Am J Roentgenol 2008; 191(1):198–206.

34. Nishie A, Yoshimitsu K, Irie H, et al. Radiologic features of Castleman's disease occupying the renal sinus. AJR Am J Roentgenol 2003;181(4):1037–40.

35. Reznek RH, Mootoosamy I, Webb JA, et al. CT in renal and perirenal lymphoma: a further look. Clin Radiol 1990;42(4):233–8.

36. Ruan J, Hyjek E, Kermani P, et al. Magnitude of stromal hemangiogenesis correlates with histologic subtype of non-Hodgkin's lymphoma. Clin Cancer Res 2006;12(19):5622–31.

37. Truong LD, Caraway N, Ngo T, et al. Renal lymphoma. The diagnostic and therapeutic roles of fine-needle aspiration. Am J Clin Pathol 2001; 115(1):18–31.

38. Heiken JP, Gold RP, Schnur MJ, et al. Computed tomography of renal lymphoma with ultrasound correlation. J Comput Assist Tomogr 1983;7(2): 245–50.

39. Herts BR, Coll DM, Novick AC, et al. Enhancement characteristics of papillary renal neoplasms revealed on triphasic helical CT of the kidneys. AJR Am J Roentgenol 2002;178(2):367–72.

40. Kim JK, Kim TK, Ahn HJ, et al. Differentiation of subtypes of renal cell carcinoma on helical CT scans. AJR Am J Roentgenol 2002;178(6): 1499–506.

41. Semelka RC, Kelekis NL, Burdeny DA, et al. Renal lymphoma: demonstration by MR imaging. AJR Am J Roentgenol 1996;166(4):823–7.

42. Oliva MR, Glickman JN, Zou KH, et al. Renal cell carcinoma: T1 and T2 signal intensity characteristics of papillary and clear cell types correlated with pathology. AJR Am J Roentgenol 2009; 192(6):1524–30.

43. Zukotynski K, Lewis A, O'Regan K, et al. PET/CT and renal pathology: a blind spot for radiologists? Part 2–lymphoma, leukemia, and metastatic disease. AJR Am J Roentgenol 2012;199(2):W168–74.

44. Kim YR, Kim JS, Min YH, et al. Prognostic factors in primary diffuse large B-cell lymphoma of adrenal gland treated with rituximab-CHOP chemotherapy from the Consortium for Improving Survival of Lymphoma (CISL). J Hematol Oncol 2012;5:49.

45. Rashidi A, Fisher SI. Primary adrenal lymphoma: a systematic review. Ann Hematol 2013;92(12): 1583–93.

46. Straus DJ, Filippa DA, Lieberman PH, et al. The non-Hodgkin's lymphomas. I. A retrospective clinical and pathologic analysis of 499 cases diagnosed between 1958 and 1969. Cancer 1983; 51(1):101–9.

47. Rosenberg SA, Diamond HD, Jaslowitz B, et al. Lymphosarcoma: a review of 1269 cases. Medicine (Baltimore) 1961;40:31–84.

48. Paling MR, Williamson BR. Adrenal involvement in non-Hodgkin lymphoma. AJR Am J Roentgenol 1983;141(2):303–5.

49. Elsayes KM, Mukundan G, Narra VR, et al. Adrenal masses: MR imaging features with pathologic correlation. Radiographics 2004;24(Suppl 1):S73–86.

50. Merklin RJ. Suprarenal gland lymphatic drainage. Am J Anat 1966;119(3):359–74.

51. Blake MA, Cronin CG, Boland GW. Adrenal imaging. AJR Am J Roentgenol 2010;194(6): 1450–60.

52. Elaini AB, Shetty SK, Chapman VM, et al. Improved detection and characterization of adrenal disease with PET-CT. Radiographics 2007;27(3):755–67.

53. Lattin GE Jr, Sturgill ED, Tujo CA, et al. From the radiologic pathology archives: Adrenal tumors and tumor-like conditions in the adult: radiologic-pathologic correlation. Radiographics 2014;34(3): 805–29.

54. Zhou L, Peng W, Wang C, et al. Primary adrenal lymphoma: radiological; pathological, clinical correlation. Eur J Radiol 2012;81(3):401–5.

55. Apter S, Avigdor A, Gayer G, et al. Calcification in lymphoma occurring before therapy: CT features and clinical correlation. AJR Am J Roentgenol 2002;178(4):935–8.

56. Paulsen SD, Nghiem HV, Korobkin M, et al. Changing role of imaging-guided percutaneous biopsy of adrenal masses: evaluation of 50 adrenal biopsies. AJR Am J Roentgenol 2004;182(4):1033–7.

57. Lokesh KN, Sathyanarayanan V, Kuntegowdanahalli CL, et al. Primary diffuse large B-cell lymphoma of testis: a single centre experience and review of literature. Urol Ann 2014;6(3): 231–4.

58. Ahmad SS, Idris SF, Follows GA, et al. Primary testicular lymphoma. Clin Oncol (R Coll Radiol) 2012;24(5):358–65.

59. Dogra VS, Gottlieb RH, Oka M, et al. Sonography of the scrotum. Radiology 2003;227(1):18–36.

60. Coursey Moreno C, Small WC, Camacho JC, et al. Testicular tumors: what radiologists need to know–differential diagnosis, staging, and management. Radiographics 2015;35(2):400–15.

61. Lantz AG, Power N, Hutton B, et al. Malignant lymphoma of the testis: a study of 12 cases. Can Urol Assoc J 2009;3(5):393–8.

62. Cheah CY, Wirth A, Seymour JF. Primary testicular lymphoma. Blood 2014;123(4):486–93.

63. Vural F, Cagirgan S, Saydam G, et al. Primary testicular lymphoma. J Natl Med Assoc 2007; 99(11):1277–82.

64. Mazloom A, Fowler N, Medeiros LJ, et al. Outcome of patients with diffuse large B-cell lymphoma of the testis by era of treatment: The M. D. Anderson Cancer Center experience. Leuk Lymphoma 2010; 51(7):1217–24.

65. Orlandini GE, Holstein AF, Moller R. Lymphatic system of the human testis. Bull Assoc Anat (Nancy) 1979;63(182):309–16 [in French].

66. Mazzu D, Jeffrey RB Jr, Ralls PW. Lymphoma and leukemia involving the testicles: findings on gray-scale and color Doppler sonography. AJR Am J Roentgenol 1995;164(3):645–7.

67. Andipa E, Liberopoulos K, Asvestis C. Magnetic resonance imaging and ultrasound evaluation of penile and testicular masses. World J Urol 2004; 22(5):382–91.

68. Tsili AC, Argyropoulou MI, Giannakis D, et al. MRI in the characterization and local staging of testicular neoplasms. AJR Am J Roentgenol 2010; 194(3):682–9.

69. Wang C, Wang H, Wang Q, et al. Primary testicular lymphoma: experience with 13 cases and literature review. Int J Hematol 2013;97(2):240–5.

70. Liu KL, Chang CC, Huang KH, et al. Imaging diagnosis of testicular lymphoma. Abdom Imaging 2006;31(5):610–2.

71. Johnson JO, Mattrey RF, Phillipson J. Differentiation of seminomatous from nonseminomatous testicular tumors with MR imaging. AJR Am J Roentgenol 1990;154(3):539–43.

72. Saito W, Amanuma M, Tanaka J, et al. A case of testicular malignant lymphoma with extension to the epididymis and spermatic cord. Magn Reson Med Sci 2002;1(1):59–63.

73. Aganovic L, Cassidy F. Imaging of the scrotum. Radiol Clin North Am 2012;50(6):1145–65.

74. Tsili AC, Argyropoulou MI, Giannakis D, et al. Primary diffuse large B-cell testicular lymphoma: magnetic resonance imaging findings. Andrologia 2012;44(Suppl 1):845–7.

75. Lagoo AS, Robboy SJ. Lymphoma of the female genital tract: current status. Int J Gynecol Pathol 2006;25(1):1–21.

76. Paladugu RR, Bearman RM, Rappaport H. Malignant lymphoma with primary manifestation in the gonad: a clinicopathologic study of 38 patients. Cancer 1980;45(3):561–71.

77. Chorlton I, Norris HJ, King FM. Malignant reticulo-endothelial disease involving the ovary as a primary manifestation: a series of 19 lymphomas and 1 granulocytic sarcoma. Cancer 1974;34(2): 397–407.

78. Vang R, Medeiros LJ, Warnke RA, et al. Ovarian non-Hodgkin's lymphoma: a clinicopathologic study of eight primary cases. Mod Pathol 2001; 14(11):1093–9.

79. Monterroso V, Jaffe ES, Merino MJ, et al. Malignant lymphomas involving the ovary. A clinicopathologic analysis of 39 cases. Am J Surg Pathol 1993;17(2): 154–70.

80. Senol T, Doger E, Kahramanoglu I, et al. Five cases of non-Hodgkin B-cell lymphoma of the ovary. Case Rep Obstet Gynecol 2014;2014:392758.

81. Horger M, Muller-Schimpfle M, Yirkin I, et al. Extensive peritoneal and omental lymphomatosis with raised CA 125 mimicking carcinomatosis: CT and intraoperative findings. Br J Radiol 2004;77(913): 71–3.

82. Dimopoulos MA, Daliani D, Pugh W, et al. Primary ovarian non-Hodgkin's lymphoma: outcome after treatment with combination chemotherapy. Gynecol Oncol 1997;64(3):446–50.

83. Chien JC, Chen CL, Chan WP. Case 210: primary ovarian lymphoma. Radiology 2014; 273(1):306–9.

84. Suzuki T, Sasano H, Takaya R, et al. Leukocytes in normal-cycling human ovaries: immunohistochemical distribution and characterization. Hum Reprod 1998;13(8):2186–91.

85. Shaaban AM, Rezvani M, Elsayes KM, et al. Ovarian malignant germ cell tumors: cellular classification and clinical and imaging features. Radiographics 2014;34(3):777–801.

86. Levine D, Brown DL, Andreotti RF, et al. Management of asymptomatic ovarian and other adnexal cysts imaged at US: Society of Radiologists in Ultrasound Consensus Conference Statement. Radiology 2010;256(3):943–54.

87. Ratner ES, Staib LH, Cross SN, et al. The clinical impact of gynecologic MRI. AJR Am J Roentgenol 2015;204(3):674–80.

88. Fox H, Langley FA, Govan AD, et al. Malignant lymphoma presenting as an ovarian tumour: a clinicopathological analysis of 34 cases. Br J Obstet Gynaecol 1988;95(4):386–90.

89. Ferrozzi F, Catanese C, Uccelli M, et al. Ovarian lymphoma. Findings with ultrasonography, computerized tomography and magnetic resonance. Radiol Med 1998;95(5):493–7 [in Italian].

90. Islimye Taskin M, Gokgozoglu L, Kandemir B. Primary ovarian large B-cell lymphoma. Case Rep Obstet Gynecol 2013;2013:493836.

91. Ferrozzi F, Tognini G, Bova D, et al. Non-Hodgkin lymphomas of the ovaries: MR findings. J Comput Assist Tomogr 2000;24(3):416–20.

92. Jung SE, Lee JM, Rha SE, et al. CT and MR imaging of ovarian tumors with emphasis on differential diagnosis. Radiographics 2002;22(6):1305–25.

93. Mitsumori A, Joja I, Hiraki Y. MR appearance of non-Hodgkin's lymphoma of the ovary. AJR Am J Roentgenol 1999;173(1):245.

94. Crawshaw J, Sohaib SA, Wotherspoon A, et al. Primary non-Hodgkin's lymphoma of the ovaries: imaging findings. Br J Radiol 2007;80(956):e155–8.

95. Harris NL, Scully RE. Malignant lymphoma and granulocytic sarcoma of the uterus and vagina. A clinicopathologic analysis of 27 cases. Cancer 1984;53(11):2530–45.

96. Kosari F, Daneshbod Y, Parwaresch R, et al. Lymphomas of the female genital tract: a study of 186 cases and review of the literature. Am J Surg Pathol 2005;29(11):1512–20.

97. Vang R, Medeiros LJ, Ha CS, et al. Non-Hodgkin's lymphomas involving the uterus: a clinicopathologic analysis of 26 cases. Mod Pathol 2000; 13(1):19–28.

98. Thyagarajan MS, Dobson MJ, Biswas A. Case report: appearance of uterine cervical lymphoma on MRI: a case report and review of the literature. Br J Radiol 2004;77(918):512–5.

99. Kim YS, Koh BH, Cho OK, et al. MR imaging of primary uterine lymphoma. Abdom Imaging 1997; 22(4):441–4.

100. Okamoto Y, Tanaka YO, Nishida M, et al. MR imaging of the uterine cervix: imaging-pathologic correlation. Radiographics 2003;23(2):425–45 [quiz: 534–5].

101. Goto N, Oishi-Tanaka Y, Tsunoda H, et al. Magnetic resonance findings of primary uterine malignant lymphoma. Magn Reson Med Sci 2007;6(1):7–13.

102. Venyo AK. Lymphoma of the urinary bladder. Adv Urol 2014;2014:327917.

103. Wong-You-Cheong JJ, Woodward PJ, Manning MA, et al. From the archives of the AFIP: neoplasms of the urinary bladder: radiologic-pathologic correlation. Radiographics 2006;26(2): 553–80.

104. Raman SP, Fishman EK. Bladder malignancies on CT: the underrated role of CT in diagnosis. AJR Am J Roentgenol 2014;203(2):347–54.

105. Martin Plata C, Rojo Todo FG, Tremps Velazquez D, et al. Primary lymphoma of the prostate: report of a clinico-pathological case and review of the literature. Actas Urol Esp 2000;24(5):437–41 [in Spanish].

106. Bostwick DG, Iczkowski KA, Amin MB, et al. Malignant lymphoma involving the prostate: report of 62 cases. Cancer 1998;83(4):732–8.

107. Chang JM, Lee HJ, Lee SE, et al. Pictorial review: Unusual tumours involving the prostate: radiological-pathological findings. Br J Radiol 2008;81(971): 907–15.

Gastrointestinal Lymphoma
Radiologic–Pathologic Correlation

Maria A. Manning, MD[a,b,*], Alexander S. Somwaru, MD[b],
Anupamjit K. Mehrotra, MD[c], Marc S. Levine, MD[d]

KEYWORDS

- Extranodal • Lymphoma • Gastrointestinal tract • Diagnosis • Imaging • Pathology

KEY POINTS

- Extranodal non-Hodgkin lymphoma is most commonly found in the gastrointestinal tract.
- The most common subtype of extranodal lymphoma found within the gastrointestinal tract is diffuse large B-cell lymphoma.
- The absence of an associated desmoplastic reaction allows these malignant lymphoid cells to expand and penetrate the wall of the gastrointestinal tract, producing characteristic radiographic findings.
- Radiologic imaging is crucial for diagnosis, staging, management, response assessment, surveillance for recurrence, and assessment of complications.

INTRODUCTION
Normal Anatomy and Histology

The gastrointestinal (GI) tract is an important component of the immune system; there are as many lymphocytes in intestinal lymphoid tissue as in the rest of the body.[1] Normal lymphoid tissue exists in varying quantities and types throughout the GI tract. Although the esophagus and stomach have minimal native mucosal lymphoid tissue, the intestines contain abundant lymphoid tissue, predominantly in the mucosa and submucosa, also known as mucosa-associated lymphoid tissue (MALT). This lymphoid tissue has an important role protecting the freely permeable intestinal mucosa against environmental antigens. Chronic antigenic stimulation or inflammation of the GI tract can lead to monoclonal proliferation in typical sites such as the distal ileum or in atypical sites such as the stomach as a response to chronic *Helicobacter pylori* gastritis. Over time, this lymphoproliferation can lead to the development of various forms of GI lymphoma.

Clinical Features

The GI tract is the most common site of extranodal lymphoma.[2–4] Although the stomach contains minimal native lymphoid tissue, it is paradoxically the most common location for extranodal lymphoma in the GI tract, followed by the small intestine (most commonly the distal ileum), colon, and

Dr M.S. Levine is a consultant for Bracco Diagnostics, Inc. The remaining authors have nothing to disclose. The views expressed in this article are those of the authors and do not necessarily reflect the official policy or position of the Department of Defense or the US Government.

[a] American Institute for Radiologic Pathology, 1010 Wayne Avenue, Suite 320, Silver Spring, MD 20910, USA; [b] Division of Abdominal Imaging, Department of Radiology, MedStar Georgetown University Hospital, 3800 Reservoir Road Northwest, Washington, DC 20007, USA; [c] The Joint Pathology Center, 606 Stephen Sitter Avenue, Silver Spring, MD 20910, USA; [d] Department of Radiology, Hospital of the University of Pennsylvania, 3400 Spruce Street, Philadelphia, PA 19104, USA
* Corresponding author. American Institute for Radiologic Pathology, 1010 Wayne Avenue, Suite 320, Silver Spring, MD 20910.
E-mail address: mmanning@acr.org

Radiol Clin N Am 54 (2016) 765–784
http://dx.doi.org/10.1016/j.rcl.2016.03.007

rectum.[3,5] GI lymphoma most commonly occurs in patients with generalized lymphoma secondarily involving the GI tract, but some patients can have primary GI lymphoma in the absence of disseminated disease. The definition of primary GI lymphoma varies among authors, but lymphomas that predominantly involve the GI tract and cause (GI) symptoms at the time of presentation are considered primary GI lymphomas, regardless of the presence or absence of lymph node involvement.[6]

There is a slight male predominance for all subtypes of lymphoma, with the exception of follicular cell lymphoma. Other than Burkitt lymphoma, which tends to affect a younger population (median age, 41 years), the majority of patients with primary GI lymphoma (>75%) present after 55 years of age (the average age at diagnosis is approximately 64 years).[3,4,7,8] When patients are symptomatic, they most commonly complain of nonspecific dysphagia or dyspepsia, vague abdominal pain, nausea and vomiting, anorexia, weight loss, and diarrhea, depending on the site of involvement.[9] Patients with more aggressive tumors may present with severe abdominal pain, a palpable mass, or acute GI perforation.[10]

Pathologic Features

Although it would be easy to consider lymphoma as a single disease with a spectrum of histologic grades, lymphomas are actually a heterogeneous group of distinct pathologic entities associated with a wide spectrum of clinical findings. These pathologic and clinical features often enable diagnosis of a specific lymphoma subtype.[11] GI lymphomas are broadly characterized by the World Health Organization as B cell or T cell, with subcategorization as precursor cell or mature cell

origins.[12] Non-Hodgkin B-cell lymphomas constitute the majority of primary GI lymphomas in the Western hemisphere. However, there is considerable geographic variation in subtype prevalence; primary GI lymphomas most commonly are diffuse large B cell or extranodal marginal zone B cell of MALT subtype in North America (**Table 1**).[3,4,7]

It is important to understand the underlying pathology and characteristic imaging appearances of the most common types of GI lymphoma, because the evaluation, diagnosis, treatment, and prognosis of these lesions are generally different from those of other, more common cancers of the GI tract.

B-CELL LYMPHOMA
Diffuse Large B-Cell Lymphoma

Diffuse large B-cell lymphoma (DLBCL), the most common form of primary GI lymphoma in adults, most commonly arises in the stomach, although it can be found throughout the GI tract.[3,4,7] DLBCL is an aggressive form of lymphoma that can arise de novo in the GI tract or from progression or transformation of indolent or low-grade small B-cell lymphoma. When DLBCL develops in the stomach, it is commonly associated with chronic H pylori infection, and up to 50% of patients have coexisting extranodal marginal zone lymphoma (ENMZL).[13,14] Major risk factors include immunodeficiency states and Epstein–Barr virus (EBV). Prognosis and survival depend on the age of the patient and the stage of the disease at the time of presentation. Progression is rapid, and, if untreated, the prognosis is poor. Nevertheless, excellent responses have been obtained using aggressive combination chemoimmunotherapy with or without concomitant radiation therapy. For a subset of patients with limited stage H pylori–related gastric DLBCL, with or without

Table 1
Gastrointestinal extranodal lymphoma by type, frequency and clinical behavior

Lymphoma Type	Frequency (%)	Clinical Behavior
Diffuse large B-cell lymphoma	47	Aggressive; curable (40%)
Extranodal marginal zone lymphoma of mucosa-associated lymphoid tissue	24	Localized; curable
Follicular lymphoma	8	Indolent- moderately aggressive; incurable
Mantle cell lymphoma	5	Moderately aggressive, bulky disease; incurable
Burkitt lymphoma	5	Aggressive; curable (90%)
Enteropathy associated T-cell lymphoma	3	Poor prognosis owing to abdominal complications

concomitant ENMZL, *H pylori* eradication therapy has shown marked clinical response, with complete regression of tumor in 50% to 80% of patients in the absence of surgery, radiation, or chemotherapy.[15,16]

Pathologic Features

DLBCL usually is manifested grossly by a mass-forming lesion, often containing areas of ulceration.[5,10,17] In most cases, there is infiltration of the bowel wall from the submucosa to the serosa, and the absence of a desmoplastic reaction often leads to penetration of the mucosa (with associated ulceration) and/or the serosa (with associated perforation) as well as frequent invasion of adjacent structures (**Fig. 1**). These tumors consist microscopically of diffuse sheets of large lymphoid cells with nuclei twice the size of normal lymphocytes infiltrating the lamina propria and destroying the normal mural architecture (**Fig. 2**). There is a moderate to high proliferation index, usually demonstrated on ki-67 stains, although this index is not as high as in Burkitt lymphoma. Immunohistochemistry can differentiate de novo DLBCL from a transformed DLBCL arising from MALT in patients with chronic *H pylori* gastritis, although the clinical behavior of these tumors is similar.[8,10]

Imaging Features

DLBCLs most commonly appear on imaging studies as large, bulky tumors, often containing areas of ulceration where the lymphomatous cells penetrate the mucosa. Barium studies typically reveal a bulky mass (often with associated areas of ulceration; **Fig. 3**), diffusely thickened folds, or circumferential narrowing, characteristically involving a long segment of bowel, without evidence of obstruction (**Fig. 4**).[9]

In patients with DLBCL involving the stomach, there usually is homogeneous, marked (ie, >1 cm) gastric wall thickening on computed tomography (CT) scan, with delayed tumoral enhancement that can be differentiated from early arterial mucosal enhancement.[18] Elsewhere in the GI tract, DLBCL usually is characterized by circumferential, homogeneous bowel wall thickening (**Fig. 5**). Because this tumor does not elicit a desmoplastic reaction, obstruction is uncommon (**Fig. 6**). The characteristic finding of aneurysmal dilation is thought to result from tumor infiltrating and weakening the muscularis propria, with destruction of the autonomic nerve plexus. Enhancement is usually homogeneous, except in the presence of necrosis, and can be quite avid in patients with more aggressive DLBCL subtypes. Ulceration and perforation can occur, and there often is bulky regional lymphadenopathy (**Fig. 7**). In the absence of perforation, however, fat planes are usually preserved.

These tumors usually are characterized on ultrasonography (US) by hypoechoic circumferential wall thickening (see **Fig. 7**). DLBCL has high fluorine-18 fluorodeoxyglucose (FDG) uptake on PET or PET/CT, which may be helpful for assessing lymph node involvement when staging these tumors (**Fig. 8**).[19] MR imaging characteristics have not been well-described, but DLBCL often is characterized by circumferential or eccentric wall thickening with homogeneous enhancement. T2 signal in these tumors usually is hyperintense in comparison with the psoas muscle.[20] Long segment involvement, aneurysmal dilation, mesenteric lymphadenopathy,

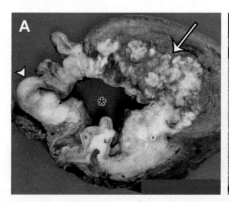
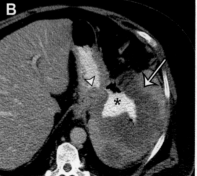

Fig. 1. Diffuse large B-cell lymphoma of the stomach. (*A*) The sectioned specimen shows a pale mass with irregular borders diffusely infiltrating the gastric wall (*arrowhead*) and extending into the spleen (*arrow*). Note central area of cavitation (*asterisk*). (*B*) Axial multidetector computed tomography image shows focal thickening of the gastric wall along the greater curvature (*arrowhead*) with associated perforation and localized extravasation of contrast into the splenic hilum (*asterisk*). Also note extension of tumor into the adjacent spleen (*arrow*).

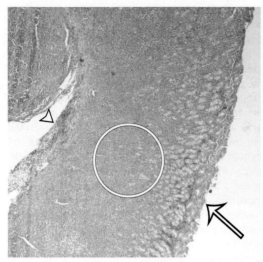

Fig. 2. Diffuse large B-cell lymphoma of the stomach. Photomicrograph (original magnification, ×4; stain: hematoxylin and eosin) of the gastric wall shows sheets of abnormal lymphocytes infiltrating the lamina propria (*circle*) with destruction of the muscularis propria and transmural extension of tumor from the mucosa (*arrow*) to the serosa (*arrowhead*).

and the absence of intestinal obstruction are other helpful features on MR imaging.[21]

Diagnostic Criteria

- Bulky disease with focal or diffuse mural infiltration and expansion.
- Homogeneous lesion with preservation of surrounding fat.
- Usually associated with bulky regional lymphadenopathy.

Differential Diagnosis

- Adenocarcinoma is much more common in the stomach and colon than DLBCL; wall thickening should be less pronounced; infiltration of the surrounding fat is common; and, when present, lymphadenopathy is less bulky.
- Infectious/inflammatory nonneoplastic entities: preserved wall stratification and the absence of lymphadenopathy are helpful features for distinguishing these benign conditions from malignant tumor.

Radiologic–Pathologic Correlation Pearls

- DLBCL is characterized by large lymphomatoid cells that infiltrate the lamina propria and expand the wall of the involved GI tract segment.
- The absence of a desmoplastic reaction often leads to penetration of the mucosa (with associated ulceration) or the serosa (with associated perforation and invasion of adjacent structures).

EXTRANODAL MARGINAL ZONE LYMPHOMA

Marginal zone lymphoma is a low-grade lymphoma arising in cells from the marginal zone surrounding lymphoid follicles. In the GI tract, ENMZL, previously known as marginal zone lymphoma of MALT (ie, MALT lymphoma), is second in frequency only to DLBCL, most commonly arising in the stomach. It has been well-documented that there is a strong association between ENMZL and *H pylori*, which has been identified in up to 90% of patients with this form of lymphoma.[22,23] Chronic *H pylori*–associated gastritis causes the formation of lymphoid follicles in the stomach, which usually is devoid of lymphoid tissue. The combined effect of specific *H pylori* strains and host immune response factors can then lead to polyclonal proliferation of malignant B cells in a perifollicular distribution from

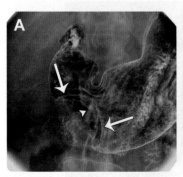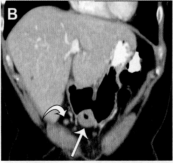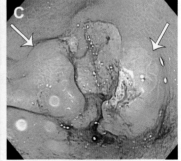

Fig. 3. Diffuse large B-cell lymphoma of the stomach. (*A*) Double-contrast spot image of the gastric antrum shows a bulky, smooth-surfaced submucosal mass (*arrows*) containing a focal area of central ulceration (*arrowhead*). (*B*) Multidetector computed tomography reformatted coronal image shows marked homogeneous circumferential wall thickening (*arrow*) with central ulceration. Also note adjacent lymphadenopathy (*curved arrow*). (*C*) Single image from an upper endoscopy confirms the presence of a nonbleeding ulcer with heaped-up margins (*arrows*), corresponding with a submucosal hypoechoic mass on endoscopic ultrasonography (not shown).

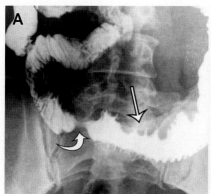
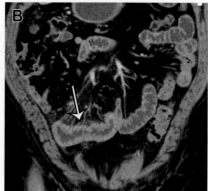

Fig. 4. Diffuse large B-cell lymphoma of the mid ileum. (*A*) Spot image from small bowel follow-through shows a focal segment of narrowing (*curved arrow*) abutting the distal end of a longer segment of nodular fold thickening in the distal ileum (*arrow*) without upstream dilation. (*B*) Coronal multidetector computed tomography image shows a long segment of homogeneous circumferential wall thickening in the distal ileum (*arrow*) without evidence of obstruction.

these reactive lymphoid follicles.[24] *H pylori* eradication therapy with antibiotics and proton pump inhibitors has resulted in sustained regression and clinical remission of these MALT lymphomas in up to 75% of patients.[23,24] Nevertheless, bulky or disseminated tumors or tumors associated with translocation t(11;18) often fail to respond to *H pylori* eradication therapy, necessitating local or systemic treatment with surgery, radiation, and/or chemotherapy.[23] Fortunately, dissemination of tumor only occurs in patients with advanced ENMZL, so affected individuals have a much better prognosis than patients with DLBCL, with an overall survival rate of 85% at 5 years.[25]

Rarely, ENMZL can involve the small bowel and colon. Immunoproliferative small intestinal disease is another type of ENMZL affecting the small bowel in young adults in the Mediterranean basin, Africa, and the Middle and Far East (previously known as

Mediterranean lymphoma or heavy chain disease).[26] This condition may be associated with chronic infection with *Campylobacter jejuni*.[27]

Pathologic Features

Gastric ENMZL is multifocal and superficial, most commonly affecting the antrum and distal body, but the entire stomach may be involved. These tumors are often manifested grossly by mucosal nodularity, thickened rugal folds, and/or ulceration.[13,28] In the small bowel, ENMZL tends to spread circumferentially, most commonly in the ileum, whereas immunoproliferative small intestinal disease preferentially affects the jejunum, causing nodular fold thickening.[13,26] Histopathologically, the tumor cells are confined to the mucosal and submucosal layers of the bowel. Lymphoid follicles are invariably present; the

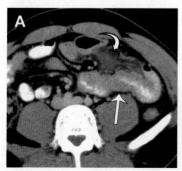
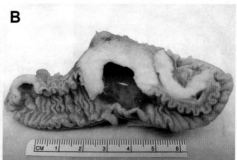

Fig. 5. Diffuse large B-cell lymphoma of the jejunum. (*A*) Axial multidetector computed tomography image shows a long segment of homogeneous, low-attenuation thickening of the small bowel wall (*arrow*), with mild luminal narrowing but no evidence of obstruction. Also note infiltration of the mesentery (*curved arrow*) without evidence of lymphadenopathy or pneumoperitoneum. (*B*) The sectioned gross specimen shows a circumferential rim of pale tan, glassy, homogeneous tumor in the small bowel wall with associated perforation.

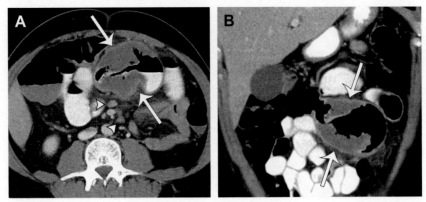

Fig. 6. Diffuse large B-cell lymphoma of the ileum. Multidetector computed tomography (*A*) axial and (*B*) coronal images show homogeneous, low-attenuation, masslike thickening of the small bowel wall (*arrows*) without luminal narrowing or evidence of obstruction. The axial image also shows subjacent lymphadenopathy (*arrowheads*).

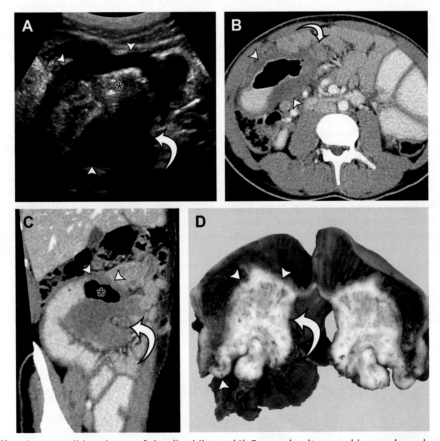

Fig. 7. Diffuse large B-cell lymphoma of the distal ileum. (*A*) Gray-scale ultrasound image shows homogeneous hypoechoic expansion of the bowel wall (*arrowheads*) surrounding a dilated gas-filled lumen (*asterisk*), with extension of hypoechoic material along the mesentery (*curved arrow*). Multidetector computed tomography (*B*) axial and (*C*) coronal oblique reconstructed images through the right upper quadrant confirm these findings, with homogeneous circumferential wall thickening of the distal ileum (*arrowheads*). Also note extension of tumor along the mesentery (*curved arrow*). (*D*) The sectioned gross specimen shows homogeneous pale tan infiltration of the wall (*arrowheads*), with extension of tumor into the mesentery (*curved arrow*).

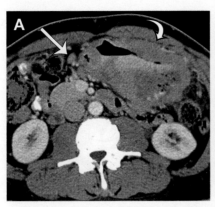
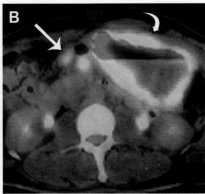

Fig. 8. Diffuse large B-cell lymphoma of the stomach. Axial (*A*) multidetector computed tomography and (*B*) PET images show homogeneous wall thickening and avid fluorine-18 fluorodeoxyglucose (FDG) uptake in the gastric antrum (*curved arrow*). FDG-avid perigastric lymph nodes (*straight arrows*) are readily identified on the PET scan.

neoplastic cells initially have a perifollicular distribution, later infiltrating the lamina propria. Tumors infiltrating the epithelium often produce characteristic lymphoepithelial lesions (**Fig. 9**). The neoplastic cells have variable morphology, consisting of a combination of monocytoid B cells, small lymphocytes, plasma cells, centroblasts, and immunoblasts.

Imaging Features

Because of the superficial nature of ENMZL involving the stomach, the findings can be extremely subtle on barium studies and are more likely to be detected on double-contrast examinations. These studies may reveal small polypoid or ulcerated lesions indistinguishable from early gastric cancers or, in other patients, focal nodularity of the mucosa, manifested by a cluster of rounded nodules of varying size that merge one with another, producing a confluent area of

disease.[27,29] Still other patients may have 1 or more ulcers or thickened rugal folds, mimicking the findings of gastritis. It therefore is important to have a low threshold for suggesting the diagnosis of ENMZL on barium studies, so endoscopy and biopsy can be obtained for a definitive diagnosis.

Cross-sectional imaging studies may reveal homogeneous mild (<1 cm), focal wall thickening, occasionally associated with small lymph nodes (see **Fig. 9**). Because mild wall thickening can be missed in an underdistended stomach, maximal distension with water or gas may facilitate detection of these lesions.[30] In the small bowel, ENMZL may be manifested by circumferential or asymmetric wall thickening (**Fig. 10**), polypoid masses, or lymphomatous polyposis, with innumerable small polyps, although the latter finding is more characteristic of mantle cell lymphoma. PET and PET/CT have a limited role in the initial evaluation of GI involvement by ENMZL because of the

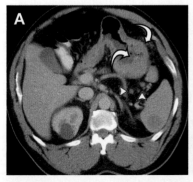
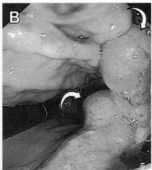
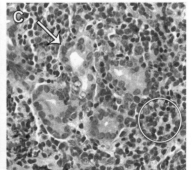

Fig. 9. Extranodal marginal zone lymphoma of the stomach. (*A*) Axial multidetector computed tomography image of the stomach shows mild homogeneous, nodular thickening of the greater curvature (*curved arrows*) with small adjacent lymph nodes (*arrowheads*). (*B*) Photograph from upper endoscopy shows the nodular, thickened folds (curved *arrows*). (*C*) Photomicrograph (original magnification ×100; stain: hematoxylin and eosin) of the specimen shows sheets of small monocytoid lymphocytes (*circle*) with lymphoepithelial lesions (*arrow*).

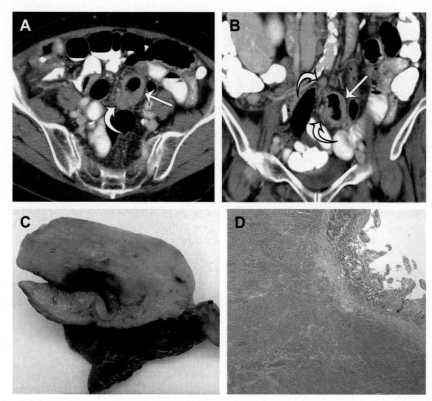

Fig. 10. Extranodal marginal zone lymphoma of the ileum. (*A*) Axial and (*B*) coronal multidetector computed tomography images show a short segment of homogeneous but asymmetric bowel wall thickening in the ileum (*arrows*) without evidence of obstruction. Small mesenteric and intermediate-level lymph nodes (*curved arrows*) are present. (*C*) The sectioned gross specimen shows homogeneous pale tan infiltration of the mucosa and submucosa. (*D*) Photomicrograph (original magnification, ×10; stain: hematoxylin and eosin) shows follicular architecture with infiltration of the mucosa and submucosa by small lymphocytes.

tumor's indolent growth pattern and background GI accumulation of FDG; however, PET and PET/CT are often used for staging of these tumors, monitoring therapeutic response, and continued assessment for possible relapse.[19,31]

Diagnostic Criteria

- Early lesions may be difficult to detect on imaging studies but double-contrast upper GI examinations may reveal coalescent mucosal nodularity, and CT may reveal mild (<1 cm) nodular fold and wall thickening with or without areas of ulceration.
- Most common in the stomach.

Differential Diagnosis

- Early gastric cancer and gastritis: endoscopic biopsy specimens are required for a definitive diagnosis.
- Gastric adenocarcinoma: more commonly associated with luminal narrowing, lymphadenopathy, and more avid FDG uptake.

Radiologic–Pathologic Correlation Pearls

- Most common in the stomach, directly associated with *H pylori* gastritis.
- Superficial spreading lesions with mucosal nodularity, mild fold and wall thickening, and ulceration are most common imaging findings as the neoplastic cells infiltrate the mucosa (lymphoepithelial lesions) and submucosa.
- Indolent tumor; most are curable with *H pylori* eradication therapy.

MANTLE CELL LYMPHOMA

Mantle cell lymphoma is a rare, aggressive subtype of lymphoma typically seen in middle-aged and elderly men. This tumor comprises up to 10% of primary GI lymphomas, but GI tract involvement is more often associated with widely disseminated nodal and extranodal disease. In fact, most patients (88%–92%) with aggressive mantle cell lymphoma have GI tract involvement at the time of diagnosis.[32,33] Surgery usually has a palliative role in patients with obstruction or intractable bleeding. Systemic chemotherapy is the treatment of choice, often followed by autologous stem cell transplant.[34] When localized, radiation therapy can also be an effective form of treatment. Regardless of treatment, the long-term prognosis for patients with mantle cell lymphoma is poor; the 5-year survival rate is only about 10%, with a median survival of 3 to 4 years.[13,35]

Pathologic Features

Mantle cell lymphoma involving the GI tract is manifested most commonly by lymphomatous polyposis, in which there is polypoid mucosal involvement of long segments of the GI tract by neoplastic lymphoid cells.[35] Affected individuals have innumerable 1 mm to 4 cm in size mucosal polyps throughout multiple portions of the GI tract, most commonly the small bowel and colon.

The polyps are composed histologically of small- to medium-sized atypical lymphoid cells with irregularly shaped nuclei and scant cytoplasm that arise from the inner mantle of lymphoid follicles. Immunohistochemistry is useful for differentiating these cells from ENMZL and follicular lymphomas. As expected, mantle cell lymphomas express B-cell antigens; detection of cyclin D1 is a highly specific marker, because overexpression results from translocation t(11;14) (q13;q32), the molecular hallmark of mantle cell lymphoma (**Fig. 11**).[36]

Imaging Features

Lymphomatous polyposis is a characteristic (although not specific) feature of mantle cell lymphoma. Barium studies typically reveal innumerable polypoid lesions (measuring ≤ 4 cm in size) throughout the small and large bowel, most frequently in the distal ileum, colon, and rectum. When seen on CT, the polyps may be manifested by nonobstructive wall thickening,[37] although the polypoid nature of these lesions may be more evident when the colon is better distended on CT colonography (see **Fig. 11**). On FDG-PET imaging, bowel involvement may be recognized by multiple curvilinear foci of increased uptake corresponding with affected small bowel or colonic loops.[38] Lymphadenopathy, which is common, is readily detected on CT and PET, because affected lymph nodes will be FDG avid. Splenomegaly is present in up to 50% of patients.[37]

Diagnostic Criteria

- Characteristic feature is lymphomatous polyposis.
- Lymphadenopathy is common.
- Splenomegaly in up to 50% of patients.

Differential Diagnosis

- Inherited polyposis syndromes are a much more common cause of multiple polyps, especially in young adults or patients with other clinical markers of the polyposis syndromes (ie, mucocutaneous pigmentation in Peutz–Jeghers syndrome and fibromatosis, osteomas, and dental anomalies in Gardner syndrome).
- Metastases are more common than primary tumors in the small bowel, resulting from hematogenous spread, local extension, or intraperitoneal seeding. Metastases can also present as multiple polypoid lesions in the bowel, but are usually larger than the lesions of mantle cell lymphoma, appearing as submucosal masses, often associated with central ulceration (ie, bull's-eye or target lesions).
- Follicular and ENMZL lymphomas can also present as lymphomatous polyposis, requiring biopsy/immunohistochemistry to differentiate from mantle cell lymphoma.

Radiologic–Pathologic Correlation Pearls

Invasion of the germinal center of the lymphoid follicles by neoplastic cells originating from the inner mantle leads to diffuse nodular proliferation, characterized by lymphomatous polyposis on imaging studies and gross specimens.

FOLLICULAR LYMPHOMA

Although follicular lymphoma is the most common nodal lymphoma in the United States, it is the least common subtype of primary GI non-Hodgkin lymphoma in adults. Similar to other subtypes, follicular lymphoma occurs predominantly in middle-aged patients but with an equal sex distribution.[3,4,39] Although follicular lymphomas can sometimes undergo transformation into DLBCL, most lesions are low-grade, slow-growing tumors that require no treatment in asymptomatic patients.

Pathologic Features

Follicular lymphoma is typically multifocal; 66% to 100% of patients with GI involvement are estimated to have multiple lesions throughout the GI tract,[40,41] although these lesions are found most commonly in the duodenum and jejunum. Similar to mantle cell lymphoma, follicular lymphoma is characterized usually by multiple small (1–2 mm in size) polypoid lesions. Rarely, small bowel involvement may be manifested by ulceration,

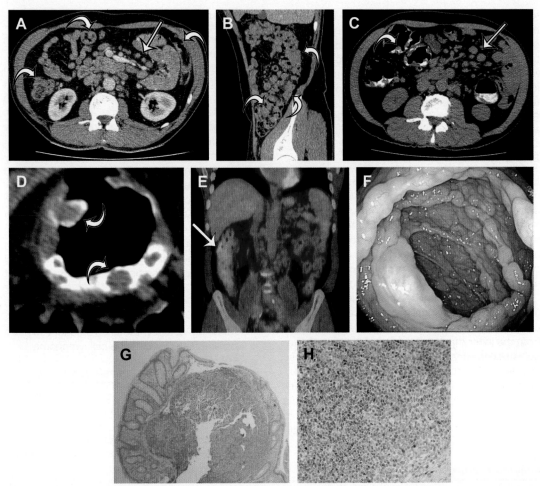

Fig. 11. Mantle cell lymphoma of the small bowel and colon. (*A*) Axial and (*B*) sagittal multidetector computed tomography (CT) images with intravenous contrast show homogeneous nodular and circumferential areas of wall thickening, most notably in the right colon, but to a lesser degree in the remaining colon (*curved arrows*), with bulky mesenteric and retroperitoneal lymphadenopathy (*arrow*). (*C, D*) Axial 2-dimensional images from CT colonography better delineate individual polypoid lesions (*curved arrows*) when luminal distention is more optimal (*Straight arrow* indicates bulky mesenteric lymphadenopathy). (*E*) Fused coronal image from PET-CT shows curvilinear uptake in the ascending colon (*arrow*). (*F*) Photograph from colonoscopy shows innumerable sessile polyps in the ascending colon. (*G*) Photomicrograph (original magnification, ×10; stain: hematoxylin and eosin) shows a lymphoid polyp with a nodular growth pattern. (*H*) Photomicrograph (original magnification, ×20; stain: cyclin D1) shows strong expression of cyclin D1.

luminal stenosis, and bulky mass lesions with or without ulceration. Polypoid lesions result from lymphomatous infiltration within intestinal villi and the development of neoplastic lymphoid follicles.[40,41]

Microscopically, small- to medium-sized lymphoid cells infiltrate the mucosa and submucosa of the duodenal and jejunal villi, forming closely packed follicles similar in size to mature germinal centers. These cells are indistinguishable from neoplastic lymphoid cells of ENMZL and mantle cell lymphoma, so immunohistochemical staining and molecular analysis are required for a definitive diagnosis.[35,40,42] Expression of CD10

enables differentiation of follicular lymphoma from ENMZL and mantle cell lymphoma.[35] Detection of translocation t(14;18) (q32;q21) is another characteristic feature.[41]

Histologic transformation to DLBCL occurs in 25% of patients with follicular lymphoma and is associated with a poor prognosis. However, such transformation has only been described in 1 case of primary GI follicular lymphoma.[41]

Imaging Features

Follicular lymphomas may be manifested on barium studies and CT by innumerable tiny polyps involving long segments of bowel, most commonly the proximal small bowel. Because of their small size, however, individual polyps frequently are not visible on imaging studies. Confluent polyps may be recognized on CT by wall thickening (**Fig. 12**).[13] Secondary features such as intestinal intussusception or associated lymphadenopathy may be the only imaging findings (**Fig. 13**). Because of the small size and relatively indolent nature of these lesions, FDG-PET is also unreliable for detection of the primary tumors, although it is useful for evaluating lymph node involvement.

Diagnostic Criteria

- Primary GI follicular lymphoma is exceedingly rare and is manifested on imaging studies by multiple tiny polypoid lesions or wall thickening.
- Better assessed by endoscopy and endoscopic ultrasonography.
- Immunohistochemistry and molecular analysis are required to differentiate from mantle cell lymphoma and ENMZL.

Differential Diagnosis

- Lymphomatous polyposis occurs more commonly in mantle cell lymphoma or ENMZL, but these lesions are typically found in the distal small bowel in mantle cell lymphoma or in the colon and stomach in ENMZL.
- Hematogenous metastasis, usually associated with widespread disease.

Radiologic–Pathologic Correlation Pearls

- Tiny polyps formed by neoplastic lymphoid follicles expanding villi.
- Slow-growing, low-grade tumor, usually confined to the lamina propria.

BURKITT LYMPHOMA

Burkitt lymphoma is a rare, highly aggressive B-cell lymphoma, considered to be the fastest growing of all malignant tumors, with a doubling time of only 24 to 48 hours. It is the most common subtype of non-Hodgkin lymphoma in children (with a peak incidence at 11 years of age), comprising up to 40% of all pediatric lymphomas,

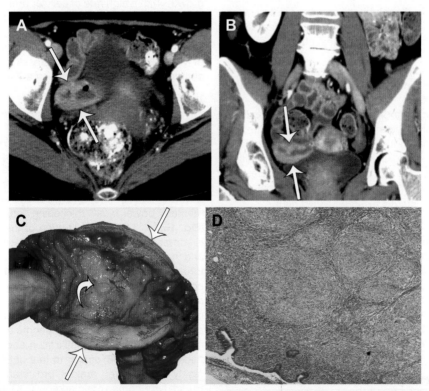

Fig. 12. Follicular lymphoma of the ileum. (*A*) Axial and (*B*) coronal multidetector computed tomography images show circumferential wall thickening in the distal ileum (*arrows*). (*C*) Intraoperative photograph of the resected specimen shows this area as a focal segment of bowel wall infiltration (*arrows*), although on close inspection, there are small nodular components (*curved arrow*). (*D*) Photomicrograph (original magnification, ×10; stain: hematoxylin and eosin) shows multiple submucosal lymphoid follicles.

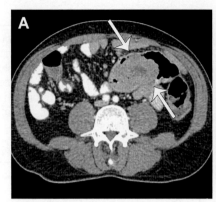
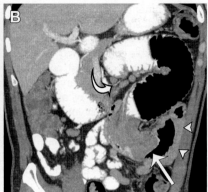

Fig. 13. Follicular lymphoma of the jejunum, causing intussusception. (*A*) Axial and (*B*) coronal multidetector computed tomography images show jejunojejunal intussusception owing to a polypoid mass (*arrows*) with separate areas of mural thickening (*arrowheads*) and mesenteric lymphadenopathy (*curved arrow*).

and is also commonly found in immunocompromised patients. Burkitt lymphoma is rare in adults (with a median age of 30 years), representing only 1% to 2% of all non-Hodgkin lymphomas and 1% to 5% of primary GI non-Hodgkin lymphomas.[43]

Burkitt lymphomas can be stratified into endemic, sporadic, and immunodeficiency-associated variants.

- Endemic lymphomas are associated with EBV; these tumors are usually found as jaw lesions in Africa and as intestinal lesions in the Middle East.
- A sporadic variant is uncommonly associated with EBV infection and commonly involves the GI tract.
- An immunodeficiency-associated variant primarily affects patients infected with the human immunodeficiency virus (HIV; up to 40% of non-Hodgkin lymphomas in HIV-positive patients are Burkitt lymphomas); these patients usually present with nodal, bony, and central nervous system involvement.[43]

Endemic Burkitt lymphoma is highly sensitive to chemotherapy, consisting of short-duration, highly intensive treatments. The 5-year survival rates exceed 90% in children with localized disease.[44] Although sporadic and immunodeficiency-associated subtypes of Burkitt lymphoma are not as chemosensitive as the endemic type, intensive chemotherapy is associated with a 50% to 70% overall survival rate in adults.[43]

Pathologic Features

Primary GI Burkitt lymphoma usually affects the terminal ileum or ileocecal region and, less commonly, the stomach or colon. There is near complete replacement of the normal gastric or bowel wall histologic architecture by diffusely spreading sheets of atypical medium-sized lymphoid cells with multiple nucleoli, basophilic cytoplasm, and numerous mitotic figures, causing extensive bowel wall thickening or a large mass.[45]

These tumors are characterized molecularly by translocation and deregulation of the c-MYC gene on chromosome 8, and they tend to undergo rapid growth, with a high rate of cellular proliferation (the index for cellular proliferation usually exceeds 99%).[45] Macrophages containing apoptotic cellular debris interspersed within dense sheets of lymphoid cells create the starry sky appearance characteristic of Burkitt lymphoma (**Fig. 14**).[8]

Imaging Features

Nonendemic Burkitt lymphoma most commonly presents with bowel involvement, typically the ileocecal region. These aggressive, rapidly proliferating cells expand the bowel folds and wall, with markedly thickened valvulae conniventes as a characteristic finding on barium studies and marked bowel wall thickening on CT scans (**Fig. 15**).[46–48] Diffuse infiltration of the bowel wall is sometimes associated with aneurysmal dilation, and the thickened walls can serve as the lead point for an intestinal intussusception (**Fig. 16**). There is commonly infiltration of the mesentery and peritoneum, with diffuse lymphadenopathy and peritoneal carcinomatosis (**Fig. 17**). When arising in the stomach or colon, Burkitt lymphoma may be manifested by submucosal infiltration and bowel wall thickening (**Fig. 18**) similar to that of DLBCL.[48] As highly aggressive, rapidly proliferating tumors, Burkitt lymphomas are markedly FDG avid at initial presentation, but show reversal of this finding with successful therapy, so FDG-PET and PET/CT scanning are useful imaging studies for initial staging and assessment of therapeutic response.

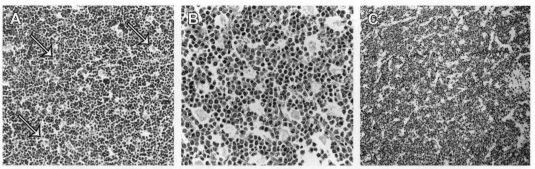

Fig. 14. Characteristic histology and immunohistochemistry of Burkitt lymphoma. (*A*) Photomicrograph (original magnification, ×20; stain: hematoxylin and eosin) at low power shows the classic starry sky appearance with macrophages (*arrows*) containing apoptotic cellular debris interspersed within dense sheets of lymphoid cells. (*B*) Photomicrograph (original magnification, ×100; stain: hematoxylin and eosin) at high power shows medium-sized lymphoid cells with squared-off nuclei, scant basophilic cytoplasm, and numerous mitotic figures. (*C*) Photomicrograph (original magnification, ×10; stain: Ki-67) shows a cellular proliferation index of more than 99%.

Diagnostic Criteria

Extranodal disease involving the bowel, particularly the ileocecal region, in a young patient with rapidly progressive symptoms should suggest Burkitt lymphoma.

Differential Diagnosis

In older patients, DLBCL should be considered as another cause for marked bowel wall thickening.

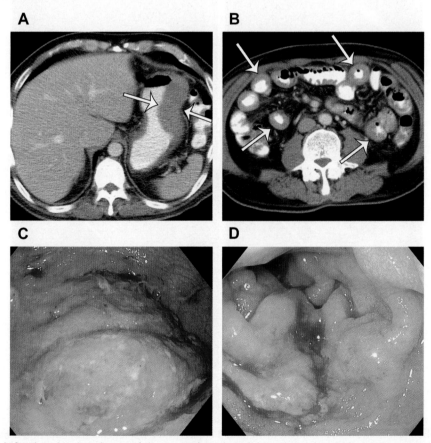

Fig. 15. Multifocal Burkitt lymphoma of the stomach and small bowel. Axial multidetector computed tomography images through the (*A*) upper and (*B*) mid abdomen show homogeneous wall thickening of the greater curvature of the stomach and multiple small bowel loops (*arrows*). Photographs from upper endoscopy show (*C*) a large nodular mass arising from the greater curvature of the gastric body with areas of ulceration and (*D*) markedly thickened folds in the duodenum.

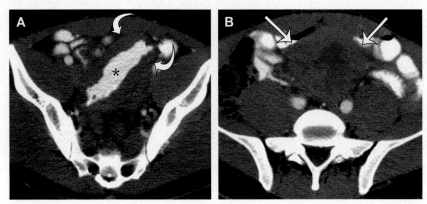

Fig. 16. Burkitt lymphoma of the ileum. (*A*, *B*) Axial multidetector computed tomography images show homogeneous, marked wall thickening of a distal small bowel loop (*curved arrows*), with aneurysmal dilation (*asterisk*) of the involved bowel. Note blurring of the serosal margins of the bowel and a contiguous heterogeneous mesenteric mass (*arrows*) within the subjacent small bowel mesentery.

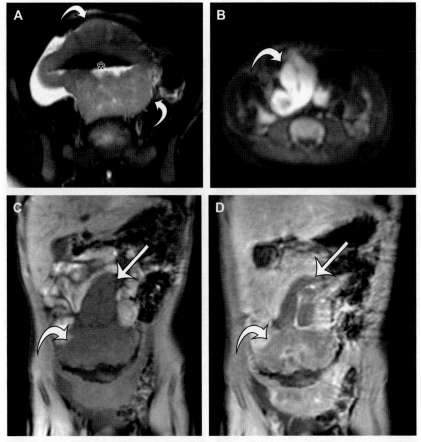

Fig. 17. Burkitt lymphoma with diffuse mesenteric spread. (*A*) Axial T2-weighted, fat-suppressed MR image of the lower abdomen shows a small amount of free fluid adjacent to a homogeneously hyperintense (relative to muscle), markedly thickened loop of small bowel (*curved arrows*) with aneurysmal dilation (*asterisk*). (*B*) Axial diffusion-weighted image shows restricted diffusion in the affected small bowel loops (*curved arrow*) owing to high cellularity. (*C*) Coronal T1-weighted fat-suppressed image shows homogeneous hypointensity of the affected small bowel loop (*curved arrow*) and infiltration of the mesentery (*arrows*). (*D*) Post gadolinium image shows mild heterogeneous enhancement.

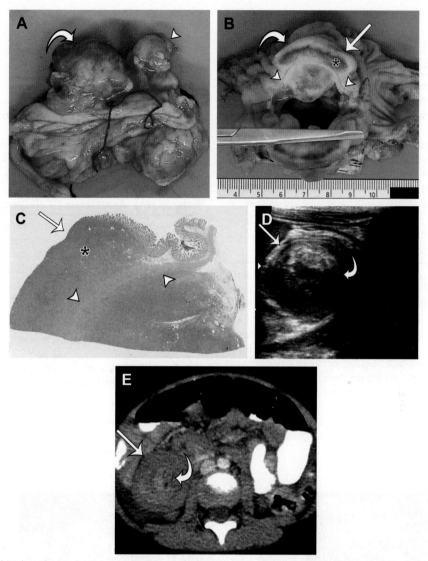

Fig. 18. Burkitt lymphoma in the ileocecal region causing intussusception. (*A*) The resected specimen shows a dominant nodular submucosal mass in the cecum (*curved arrow*) and a smaller submucosal mass at the ileocecal valve (*arrowhead*). (*B*) The larger mass (*curved arrow*) after sectioning shows a nodular, white-tan mass with areas of hemorrhage (*asterisk*) encasing the muscularis propria (*arrowheads*) beneath an intact mucosa (*arrow*). (*C*) Photomicrograph (original magnification, 4; stain: hematoxylin and eosin) shows diffuse lymphoid infiltration of the bowel wall. (*Arrow* indicates the mucosal surface, *arrowheads* indicate muscularis propria, and *asterisk* indicates area of hemorrhage. Note how the findings correlate with those on the cut specimen.) (*D*) Gray-scale ultrasound image of the right lower quadrant in the transverse plane and (*E*) axial multidetector computed tomography shows the characteristic target sign associated with intussusception (*arrows*); the curved arrow (*D*, *E*) indicates the lead point, correlating with the polypoid mass shown on the gross specimen.

Radiologic–Pathologic Correlation Pearls

Highly aggressive, rapidly proliferating neoplastic B cells infiltrate the bowel wall (most commonly the small bowel or ileocecal region), causing marked fold and wall thickening, mesenteric infiltration, and lymphadenopathy; widespread disease at the time of presentation.

HODGKIN LYMPHOMA

Primary GI Hodgkin lymphoma is rare and has only been described in anecdotal case reports.[39] GI involvement is more commonly secondary to extension of tumor from adjacent lymph nodes of any Hodgkin lymphoma subtype, including nodular sclerotic, mixed cellularity, and lymphocyte-rich or lymphocyte-depleted forms.[39]

Pathologic Features

Reported cases of primary GI Hodgkin lymphoma have predominantly involved the stomach, although this tumor has been reported throughout the GI tract.[8] The most common appearance in the stomach is an infiltrating lesion, occasionally associated with areas of ulceration.[49,50] Histologically, binucleated Reed–Sternberg cells are characteristic of this form of lymphoma. Immunohistochemistry is a useful adjunct, and EBV is commonly positive.

Imaging Features

Imaging studies may show infiltration of the folds and wall of the bowel, with ulceration best appreciated on barium studies. Cross-sectional imaging studies (ultrasonography, CT, and MR imaging) may demonstrate circumferential bowel wall thickening (**Fig. 19**). It should be noted that focal stenosis and obstruction are more common in GI Hodgkin lymphoma than in GI non-Hodgkin lymphoma because of the desmoplastic reaction incited by these tumors.[49,50] FDG-PET may show increased uptake in patients with GI Hodgkin lymphoma, because these tumors are FDG avid.[51]

Diagnostic Criteria

- Extremely rare; nonspecific wall thickening.
- Reed–Sternberg cells and immunohistochemistry required for diagnosis.

Differential Diagnosis

- DLBCL and ENMZL are more common and may have similar features.
- Adenocarcinoma, especially in cases with associated stenosis and obstruction.

T-CELL LYMPHOMA
Enteropathy-Associated T-Cell Lymphoma

T-cell lymphomas constitute only 3% of all primary GI non-Hodgkin lymphomas.[3,4] The most common is enteropathy-associated T-cell lymphoma (EATL), which occurs primarily in middle-aged men (6th decade, male predominant) and is subdivided into 2 distinct types.

- Type I EATL comprises 80% to 90% of cases; strongly associated with celiac disease; and
- Type II EATL (or monomorphic CD56+ intestinal lymphoma): unrelated to celiac disease.

Both types of EATL have a poor prognosis. Intestinal perforation is a frequent complication, occurring in up to 50% of patients.[52] Patients with celiac disease are not only at increased risk

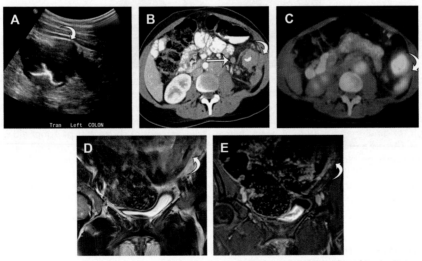

Fig. 19. Hodgkin's lymphoma of the colon. (*A*) Transverse ultrasound and (*B*) axial computed tomography images of the left colon show homogeneous circumferential wall thickening with peritoneal nodularity (*curved arrows*) and mesenteric adenopathy (*straight arrow*). (*C*) Axial PET image shows avid fluorodeoxyglucose uptake in the colon and peritoneal nodularity (*curved arrow*). Coronal (*D*) T2-weighted and (*E*) T1-weighted post gadolinium images in the pelvis show homogeneously hyperintense wall thickening and mild heterogeneous enhancement (*curved arrows*). (*Courtesy of* Dan Swerdlow, MD, Department of Radiology, MedStar Georgetown University Hospital, Washington, DC.)

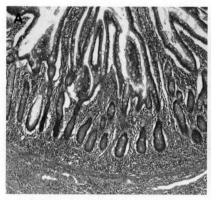
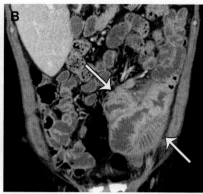

Fig. 20. Enteropathy-associated T-cell lymphoma of the jejunum, type 1. (*A*) Photomicrograph (original magnification, ×10; stain: hematoxylin and eosin) of the resected bowel shows a dense lymphoid infiltrate involving the lamina propria and submucosa. (*B*) Contrast-enhanced computed tomography in the coronal plane shows nodular jejunal wall thickening and infiltration of the mesenteric fat (*arrows*).

for developing primary malignant tumors of the GI tract, but also non-Hodgkin lymphoma, most commonly primary extranodal T-cell lymphoma of the GI tract.[53,54] Patients with refractory celiac disease or those on a 12-month gluten-free diet with aberrant intraepithelial lymphocytes are at greatest risk; as many as 60% of patients with aberrant intraepithelial lymphocytes develop EATL within 5 years.[53,54]

Pathologic Features

Type I EATL commonly affects the jejunum or proximal ileum. Type 1 EATL cells are predominantly large cells with angulated nuclei that express the HLADQ2 or HLADQ8 genotypes found in almost all patients with celiac disease. Grossly, these cells are centered on the mucosa and infiltrate the wall, forming multiple nodules or a large deeply ulcerating mass (**Fig. 20**).[54,55] Transmural invasion and necrosis lead to a high perforation rate. As expected, these patients also have

evidence of underlying celiac disease, with crypt hyperplasia, villous atrophy, and intraepithelial lymphocytosis.

In contrast, type II EATL tends to involve the distal ileum, ileocecal region, or colon.[54,55] Type II EATL cells are more uniform monotonous small or intermediate-sized cells with hyperchromatic nuclei, which are CD56 positive (whereas type I cells are CD56 negative) and have HLADQ2 or HLADQ8 frequencies comparable to those in the general population. Patients with these tumors may also have an underlying enteropathy.

Imaging Features

EATL is characterized on barium studies by thickened, nodular folds, ulcers, and strictures. CT and MR imaging studies most commonly reveal smooth circumferential wall thickening of the affected small bowel (**Fig. 21**). GI perforation is more likely to occur in patients with small bowel

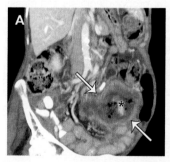
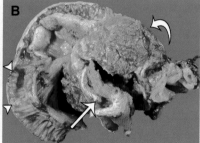
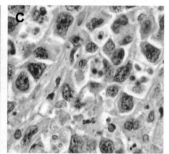

Fig. 21. Enteropathy-associated T-cell lymphoma of the jejunum, type 1. (*A*) Contrast-enhanced computed tomography reconstructed in the coronal oblique plane shows aneurysmal dilation (*asterisk*) and circumferential wall thickening of a small bowel loop in the left lower quadrant (*arrows*). (*B*) The sectioned gross specimen shows nodular wall thickening (*arrowheads*), with focal dilated segment and tumor (*curved arrow*) extending to the mucosal and serosal surfaces (*straight arrow*). (*C*) Photomicrograph (original magnification, ×400; stain: hematoxylin and eosin) shows intermediate to large lymphocytes with irregular angulated nuclei, vesicular chromatin, occasionally prominent nucleoli, and moderate amounts of eosinophilic cytoplasm.

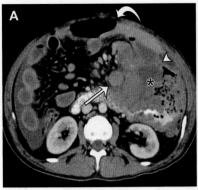 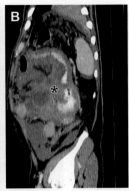 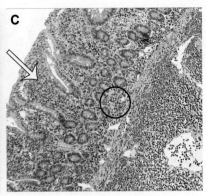

Fig. 22. Enteropathy-associated T-cell lymphoma of the jejunum, type 2. (A) Axial and (B) sagittal contrast-enhanced multidetector computed tomography images show marked heterogeneous wall thickening of the proximal jejunum (*asterisk*), with focal aneurysmal dilation, mesenteric infiltration (*arrow*) and associated perforation (*arrowhead*). Note gas and contrast (*curved arrow*). (C) Photomicrograph (original magnification, ×20; stain: hematoxylin and eosin) shows submucosal (*black circle*) and intraepithelial (*white arrow*) infiltration of bowel wall by monotonous lymphoid cells. Also note villous atrophy (around *white arrow*) and crypt hyperplasia (around *black circle*) from associated celiac enteropathy.

disease (**Fig. 22**). Patients with refractory celiac disease often have a decreased number of jejunal folds, longer segments of small bowel wall thickening, transient intussusceptions, aneurysmal dilation, infiltration of the mesenteric fat, lymphadenopathy, and splenic atrophy.[20,56,57] EATL can be differentiated from refractory celiac disease by increased uptake on FDG-PET, which occurs in 86% to 100% of patients.[55]

Diagnostic Criteria

- Thickened, nodular folds with frequent ulceration and strictures.
- Eccentric circumferential wall thickening with long-segment involvement; perforation is not uncommon.
- Ancillary findings of celiac disease, including decreased jejunal folds, aneurysmal dilation, and infiltration of the mesenteric fat.

Differential Diagnosis

- Ulcerative jejunitis: some consider this condition to be a low-grade form of EATL, but others believe it is a rare complication of celiac disease.
- Other lymphomas, including DLBCL, although T-cell lymphoma more commonly affects the proximal small bowel and is more likely to be associated with multifocal disease and a higher frequency of perforation than B-cell lymphoma.
- Inflammatory bowel disease (Crohn's disease) or infectious colitis (typically opportunistic infections in immunocompromised hosts).

- Adenocarcinoma (usually short segment disease with stricturing) or metastases in patients with widespread disease.

Radiologic–Pathologic Correlation Pearls

- Mucosally centered malignant lymphoid aggregates forming multiple mural nodules.
- Transmural infiltration expands the wall (circumferential wall thickening) and can extend to the mucosa (with ulceration) or the serosa (with perforation).

SUMMARY

GI lymphomas are a heterogeneous group of neoplasms that vary in cell lineage and biologic behavior. A multifactorial approach that includes histologic, immunohistochemical, and genetic findings is crucial for proper diagnosis and classification of GI lymphomas because of their overlapping pathologic features. Identification of key features, including the site of GI involvement, imaging findings, and associated complications, combined with the patient's clinical history and presentation, may facilitate diagnosis of the various forms of GI lymphoma and suggest the underlying histologic subtype in individual patients.

REFERENCES

1. Murphy KM. Janeway's immunobiology. 8th edition. New York: Garland Science; Taylor & Francis Group, LLC; 2011. p. 888.
2. Crump M, Gospodarowicz M, Shepherd FA. Lymphoma of the gastrointestinal tract. Semin Oncol 1999;26(3):324–37.

3. Howell JM, Auer-Grzesiak I, Zhang J, et al. Increasing incidence rates, distribution and histological characteristics of primary gastrointestinal non-Hodgkin lymphoma in a North American population. Can J Gastroenterol 2012;26(7):452–6.

4. Warrick J, Luo J, Robirds D, et al. Gastrointestinal lymphomas in a North American population: clinicopathologic features from one major Central-Midwestern United States tertiary care medical center. Diagn Pathol 2012;7:76.

5. Peng JC, Zhong L, Ran ZH. Primary lymphomas in the gastrointestinal tract. J Dig Dis 2015;16(4): 169–76.

6. Krol AD, le Cessie S, Snijder S, et al. Primary extra-nodal non-Hodgkin's lymphoma (NHL): the impact of alternative definitions tested in the Comprehensive Cancer Centre West population-based NHL registry. Ann Oncol 2003;14(1):131–9.

7. Cardona DM, Layne A, Lagoo AS. Lymphomas of the gastro-intestinal tract - pathophysiology, pathology, and differential diagnosis. Indian J Pathol Microbiol 2012;55(1):1–16.

8. Bautista-Quach MA, Ake CD, Chen M, et al. Gastrointestinal lymphomas: morphology, immunophenotype and molecular features. J Gastrointest Oncol 2012;3(3):209–25.

9. Levine MS, Rubesin SE, Pantongrag-Brown L, et al. Non-Hodgkin's lymphoma of the gastrointestinal tract: radiographic findings. AJR Am J Roentgenol 1997;168(1):165–72.

10. Nakamura S, Muller-Hermelink HK, Delabie J, et al. Lymphoma of the stomach. In: Bosman FT, Carneiro F, Hruban R, et al, editors. WHO classification of tumors of the digestive system. 4th ed. Lyon, France: International Agency for Research on Cancer; 2010. p. 69–73.

11. Jaffe ES, Harris NL, Stein H, et al. Classification of lymphoid neoplasms: the microscope as a tool for disease discovery. Blood 2008;112(12):4384–99.

12. Swerdlow SH. Lymphoma classification and the tools of our trade: an introduction to the 2012 USCAP long course. Mod Pathol 2013;26(Suppl 1): S1–14.

13. Lewis RB, Mehrotra AK, Rodríguez P, et al. From the radiologic pathology archives: gastrointestinal lymphoma: radiologic and pathologic findings. Radiographics 2014;34(7):1934–53.

14. Zullo A, Hassan C, Andriani A, et al. Primary low-grade and high-grade gastric MALT-lymphoma presentation. J Clin Gastroenterol 2010;44(5):340–4.

15. Chen LT, Lin JT, Tai JJ, et al. Long-term results of anti-Helicobacter pylori therapy in early-stage gastric high-grade transformed MALT lymphoma. J Natl Cancer Inst 2005;97(18):1345–53.

16. Ferreri AJ, Govi S, Raderer M, et al. Helicobacter pylori eradication as exclusive treatment for limited-stage gastric diffuse large B-cell lymphoma:

17. Hatano B, Ohshima K, Tsuchiya T, et al. Clinico-pathological features of gastric B-cell lymphoma: a series of 317 cases. Pathol Int 2002;52(11): 677–82.

18. Chen CY, Jaw TS, Wu DC, et al. MDCT of giant gastric folds: differential diagnosis. AJR Am J Roentgenol 2010;195(5):1124–30.

19. Paes FM, Kalkanis DG, Sideras PA, et al. FDG PET/CT of extranodal involvement in non-Hodgkin lymphoma and Hodgkin disease. Radiographics 2010;30(1):269–91.

20. Lohan DG, Alhajeri AN, Cronin CG, et al. MR enterography of small-bowel lymphoma: potential for suggestion of histologic subtype and the presence of underlying celiac disease. AJR Am J Roentgenol 2008;190(2):287–93.

21. Masselli G, Colaiacomo MC, Marcelli G, et al. MRI of the small-bowel: how to differentiate primary neoplasms and mimickers. Br J Radiol 2012;85(1014): 824–37.

22. Wotherspoon AC, Doglioni C, Diss TC, et al. Regression of primary low-grade B-cell gastric lymphoma of mucosa-associated lymphoid tissue type after eradication of Helicobacter pylori. Lancet 1993; 342(8871):575–7.

23. Ruskone-Fourmestraux A, Fischbach W, Aleman BM, et al. EGILS consensus report. Gastric extranodal marginal zone B-cell lymphoma of MALT. Gut 2011; 60(6):747–58.

24. Farinha P, Gascoyne RD. Helicobacter pylori and MALT lymphoma. Gastroenterology 2005;128(6): 1579–605.

25. Neumeister P, Troppan K, Raderer M. Management of gastric mucosa-associated lymphoid tissue lymphoma. Dig Dis 2015;33(1):11–8.

26. Vessal K, Dutz W, Kohout E, et al. Immunoproliferative small intestinal disease with duodenojejunal lymphoma: radiologic changes. AJR Am J Roentgenol 1980;135(3):491–7.

27. Foster LH, Portell CA. The role of infectious agents, antibiotics, and antiviral therapy in the treatment of extranodal marginal zone lymphoma and other low-grade lymphomas. Curr Treat Options Oncol 2015;16(6):28.

28. Kim YH, Lim HK, Han JK, et al. Low-grade gastric mucosa-associated lymphoid tissue lymphoma: correlation of radiographic and pathologic findings. Radiology 1999;212(1):241–8.

29. Yoo CC, Levine MS, Furth EE, et al. Gastric mucosa-associated lymphoid tissue lymphoma: radiographic findings in six patients. Radiology 1998;208(1):239–43.

30. Horton KM, Fishman EK. Current role of CT in imaging of the stomach. Radiographics 2003; 23(1):75–87.

31. Radan L, Fischer D, Bar-Shalom R, et al. FDG avidity and PET/CT patterns in primary gastric lymphoma. Eur J Nucl Med Mol Imaging 2008;35(8): 1424–30.

32. Romaguera JE, Medeiros LJ, Hagemeister FB, et al. Frequency of gastrointestinal involvement and its clinical significance in mantle cell lymphoma. Cancer 2003;97(3):586–91.

33. Salar A, Juanpere N, Bellosillo B, et al. Gastrointestinal involvement in mantle cell lymphoma: a prospective clinic, endoscopic, and pathologic study. Am J Surg Pathol 2006;30(10):1274–80.

34. Kluin-Nelemans HC, Hoster E, Hermine O, et al. Treatment of older patients with mantle-cell lymphoma. N Engl J Med 2012;367(6):520–31.

35. Kodama T, Ohshima K, Nomura K, et al. Lymphomatous polyposis of the gastrointestinal tract, including mantle cell lymphoma, follicular lymphoma and mucosa-associated lymphoid tissue lymphoma. Histopathology 2005;47(5):467–78.

36. Vose JM. Mantle cell lymphoma: 2015 update on diagnosis, risk-stratification, and clinical management. Am J Hematol 2015;90(8):739–45.

37. Chung HH, Kim YH, Kim JH, et al. Imaging findings of mantle cell lymphoma involving gastrointestinal tract. Yonsei Med J 2003;44(1):49–57.

38. Sam JW, Levine MS, Farner MC, et al. Detection of small bowel involvement by mantle cell lymphoma on F-18 FDG positron emission tomography. Clin Nucl Med 2002;27(5):330–3.

39. Nakamura S, Matsumoto T, Iida M, et al. Primary gastrointestinal lymphoma in Japan: a clinicopathologic analysis of 455 patients with special reference to its time trends. Cancer 2003;97(10):2462–73.

40. Yamamoto S, Nakase H, Yamashita K, et al. Gastrointestinal follicular lymphoma: review of the literature. J Gastroenterol 2010;45(4):370–88.

41. Iwamuro M, Kondo E, Takata K, et al. Diagnosis of follicular lymphoma of the gastrointestinal tract: a better initial diagnostic workup. World J Gastroenterol 2016;22(4):1674–83.

42. Shia J, Teruya-Feldstein J, Pan D, et al. Primary follicular lymphoma of the gastrointestinal tract: a clinical and pathologic study of 26 cases. Am J Surg Pathol 2002;26(2):216–24.

43. Ferry JA. Burkitt's lymphoma: clinicopathologic features and differential diagnosis. Oncologist 2006; 11(4):375–83.

44. Karantanis D, Durski JM, Lowe VJ, et al. 18F-FDG PET and PET/CT in Burkitt's lymphoma. Eur J Radiol 2010;75(1):e68–73.

45. Vade A, Blane CE. Imaging of Burkitt lymphoma in pediatric patients. Pediatr Radiol 1985;15(2):123–6.

46. Alford BA, Coccia PF, L'Heureux PR. Roentgenographic features of American Burkitt's lymphoma. Radiology 1977;124(3):763–70.

47. Johnson KA, Tung K, Mead G, et al. The imaging of Burkitt's and Burkitt-like lymphoma. Clin Radiol 1998;53(11):835–41.

48. Kamona AA, El-Khatib MA, Swaidan MY, et al. Pediatric Burkitt's lymphoma: CT findings. Abdom Imaging 2007;32(3):381–6.

49. Guermazi A, Brice P, de Kerviler EE, et al. Extranodal Hodgkin disease: spectrum of disease. Radiographics 2001;21(1):161–79.

50. Libson E, Mapp E, Dachman AH. Hodgkin's disease of the gastrointestinal tract. Clin Radiol 1994;49(3): 166–9.

51. Tsukamoto N, Kojima M, Hasegawa M, et al. The usefulness of (18)F-fluorodeoxyglucose positron emission tomography ((18)F-FDG-PET) and a comparison of (18)F-FDG-pet with (67)gallium scintigraphy in the evaluation of lymphoma: relation to histologic subtypes based on the World Health Organization classification. Cancer 2007;110(3): 652–9.

52. Byun JH, Ha HK, Kim AY, et al. CT findings in peripheral T-cell lymphoma involving the gastrointestinal tract. Radiology 2003;227(1):59–67.

53. Gale J, Simmonds PD, Mead GM, et al. Enteropathy-type intestinal T-cell lymphoma: clinical features and treatment of 31 patients in a single center. J Clin Oncol 2000;18(4):795–803.

54. Smedby KE, Akerman M, Hildebrand H, et al. Malignant lymphomas in coeliac disease: evidence of increased risks for lymphoma types other than enteropathy-type T cell lymphoma. Gut 2005;54(1): 54–9.

55. van de Water JM, Cillessen SA, Visser OJ, et al. Enteropathy associated T-cell lymphoma and its precursor lesions. Best Pract Res Clin Gastroenterol 2010;24(1):43–56.

56. Hadithi M, Mallant M, Oudejans J, et al. 18F-FDG PET versus CT for the detection of enteropathy-associated T-cell lymphoma in refractory celiac disease. J Nucl Med 2006;47(10):1622–7.

57. Mallant M, Hadithi M, Al-Toma AB, et al. Abdominal computed tomography in refractory coeliac disease and enteropathy associated T-cell lymphoma. World J Gastroenterol 2007;13(11):1696–700.

Primary Musculoskeletal Lymphoma

Mark D. Murphey, MD[a],*, Mark J. Kransdorf, MD[b]

KEYWORDS

- Extranodal lymphoma • Primary bone lymphoma • B-cell lymphoma
- Primary soft tissue lymphoma

KEY POINTS

- Primary musculoskeletal lymphoma is rare, almost invariably B cell, but often reveals imaging characteristics suggestive of the diagnosis.
- Primary osseous lymphoma shows aggressive bone destruction with soft tissue involvement, and intervening cortical destruction may be subtle.
- Primary soft tissue lymphoma typically demonstrates long cones of involvement, which may be multiple and intramuscular or intermuscular in location by MR imaging.
- PET with fluorodeoxyglucose fluorine 18 imaging reveals marked increased radionuclide uptake in areas of musculoskeletal lymphomatous involvement and is useful to evaluate disease extent, treatment effect, and recurrence.
- Initial biopsy of musculoskeletal lymphoma may suggest nondiagnostic tissue owing to discohesive and collapsed cells. However, immunohistochemical stains often remain positive, if performed.

MUSCULOSKELETAL LYMPHOMA
Introduction

Primary lymphoma of the musculoskeletal system is rare. Involvement may include the bone, subcutaneous tissue as well as muscle. Regional lymph nodes may also be affected. Imaging of primary musculoskeletal lymphoma often reveals suggestive intrinsic and morphologic features of this disease. Biopsy confirmation is vital to differentiate musculoskeletal lymphoma from sarcoma because treatment dramatically differs between these diseases. Musculoskeletal lymphoma is treated medically with overall excellent response as opposed to surgical treatment of sarcoma often supplemented with adjuvant chemotherapy and radiation therapy.

LYMPHOMA OF BONE

Primary lymphoma of bone accounts for less than 5% of malignant bone tumors.[1–3] The vast majority of cases are non-Hodgkin lymphoma. Primary Hodgkin lymphoma of the musculoskeletal system is exceedingly rare. Imaging features of skeletal lymphoma may be nonspecific and similar to other small round blue cell tumors. However, intrinsic characteristics and the morphologic appearance may reveal suggestive features.

Primary lymphoma of bone shows a wide age range of distribution with patients most commonly affected in the third and sixth through eighth decades.[1–4] There is a male predilection, with a large series by Mulligan and Kransdorf[1] showing a 1:8:1 ratio.[2,4] Long bones (71%) are affected more commonly than flat bones (22%).[1,2,4] The most commonly involved sites include the femur (33%), tibia (20%), humerus (13%), pelvis (11%), scapula (4%), clavicle (3%), ribs (3%), vertebral column (5%), foot (2%), radius (1%), and the patella (1%).[1,2,4] The specific most frequent locations are the distal femoral metadiaphysis (16%),

[a] American Institute for Radiologic Pathology (AIRP), 1010 Wayne Avenue, Suite 320, Silver Spring, MD 20910, USA; [b] Department of Radiology, Mayo Clinic Hospital, 5777 East Mayo Boulevard, Phoenix, AZ 85054, USA
* Corresponding author.
E-mail address: mmurphey@acr.org

Radiol Clin N Am 54 (2016) 785–795
http://dx.doi.org/10.1016/j.rcl.2016.03.008
0033-8389/16/$ – see front matter © 2016 Elsevier Inc. All rights reserved.

proximal metaphysis of the tibia (12%), and the femoral midshaft (8%).[1,2,4] Ephiphyseal centered lesions accounted for only 5% of cases in the series by Mulligan and Kransdorf.[1,2,4,5]

The clinical presentation of primary osseous lymphoma is frequently insidious with intermittent pain persisting for several months. Additional symptoms include swelling, palpable mass, and systemic signs, such as weight loss and fever. Vertebral lesions can result in neurologic symptoms owing to paraspinal extension.

The radiographic appearance of primary musculoskeletal lymphoma is most commonly aggressive bone destruction seen in 70% of cases[1,2,4,6] (Figs. 1–3). The pattern of bone lysis

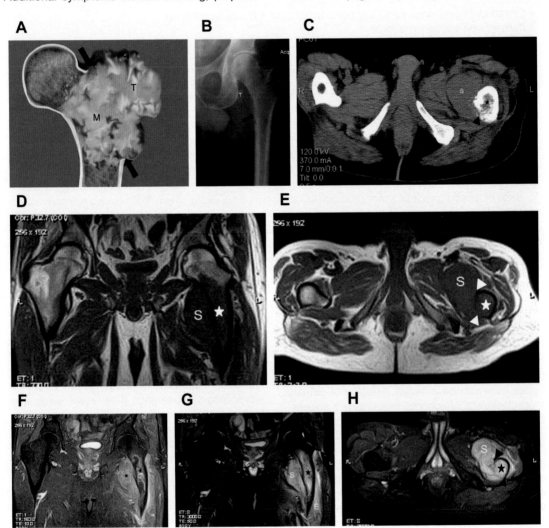

Fig. 1. Lymphoma of the proximal femur with pathologic fracture and associated soft tissue mass. (A) Pictorial representation of intramedullary lymphoma (M) with cortical destruction (arrows) and direct extensive into the soft tissue (T). (B) Frontal radiograph of the right hip shows aggressive bone destruction with cortical permeation medially (arrow) and avulsion of the lesser trochanter (T). (C) Axial CT demonstrates marrow involvement (star) with cortical destruction (arrowhead) and soft tissue extension (S). The soft tissue component has similar attenuation to muscle. (D, E) Coronal and axial T1-weighted (TR = 330; echo time [TE] = 10) MR images show marrow replacement (star) and soft tissue mass (S) in direct continuity with intervening cortical destruction (arrowheads). (F) Postcontrast fat-suppressed T1-weighted (TR = 583; TE = 10) MR image reveals mild diffuse enhancement of both the intraosseous and the soft tissue components (stars). (G, H) Coronal and axial fat-suppressed T2-weighted (TR = 3000; TE = 50) MR images demonstrate similar features with the marrow replacement (star) and soft tissue mass (S) and continuity through cortical destruction (arrowheads). The signal of the lymphomatous involvement is high intensity. There is surrounding soft tissue edema (E). ([A] From Murphey MD, Senchak LT, Mambalam PK, et al. From the radiologic pathology archives: Ewing sarcoma family of tumors: radiologic-pathologic correlation. Radiographics 2013;33(3):803–31; with permission.)

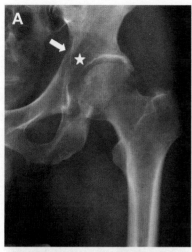

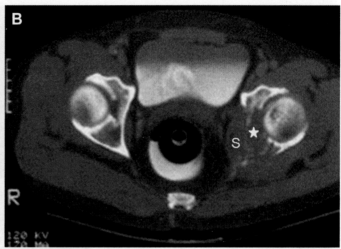

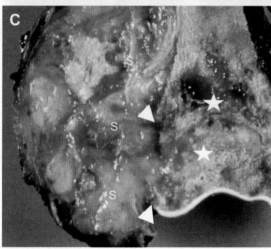

Fig. 2. Acetabular bone destruction with soft tissue mass in a 70- year-old man with primary lymphoma of bone. (*A*) Frontal hip radiograph shows aggressive bone lysis (*star*) with destruction of the iliopectineal cortex (*arrow*). (*B*) Axial CT also reveals aggressive bone lysis (*star*), cortical destruction, and associated soft tissue mass (S) in direct continuity. (*C*) Sectioned gross specimen demonstrates identical features compared with imaging with medullary involvement (*stars*), cortical destruction (*arrowhead*), and associated soft tissue mass (S) in direct continuity.

is most frequently "moth-eaten" to permeative, typical of small round blue cell tumors.[1,2,4,7] A nonaggressive radiographic appearance is only rarely reported.[8] A mixed lytic and blastic pattern is apparent in 28% of cases, and sclerosis predominates in only 2% of patients.[1,2,4] Radiographs may demonstrate normal findings in 5% of cases[1,2,4] (Fig. 4). Periosteal reaction is seen in 47% of all patients and 47% of cases affecting long bones.[1,2,4] The periosteal reaction is typically aggressive in appearance, most frequently interrupted single or multiple layers. Cortical destruction with an associated soft tissue mass can be seen on radiographs in primary osseous lymphoma in 48% of cases[1,2,4] (see Figs. 1 and 2). Additional radiographic findings include pathologic fracture at presentation in 22% of patients (see Fig. 1) and areas of sequestra-like regions in 6.5% of patients[1,2,4] (Fig. 5). In the authors' experience, areas of sclerosis are seen almost exclusively in the intraosseous

component of the lesion and represent reactive osteoid. Areas of calcification in the soft tissue component are exceedingly unusual before the initiation of treatment. Rarely, lymphoma has been described occurring on the surface of bone simulating periosteal osteosarcoma.[9,10]

Bone scintigraphy usually depicts marked increased uptake of radionuclide in 64% of cases[1,2] (see Fig. 4; Fig. 6). Mild to moderate activity is seen in 34% of patients, and normal uptake is rare (2%).[1,2,4] Similar to other areas of lymphomatous involvement, PET with fluorodeoxyglucose fluorine 18 (FDG-PET) reveals intense areas of increased radionuclide activity in primary musculoskeletal lymphoma[11–15] (see Fig. 6). FDG-PET imaging is the optimal radiologic modality to evaluate lesion multiplicity, extent of disease and response to therapy.[11]

Cross-sectional imaging (computed tomography [CT] and magnetic resonance [MR]) of

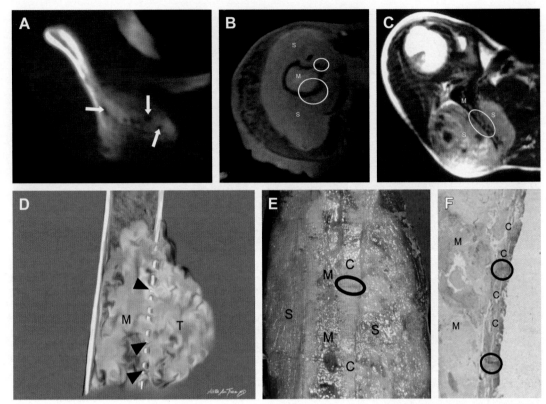

Fig. 3. Multiple examples in different patients with osseous lymphoma and permeation of the cortex allowing connection between the intraosseous and extraosseous components. (*A*) Axial CT of the scapula shows multiple small areas of cortical permeation (*arrows*). (*B, C*) Axial proton density of the humerus (TR = 1500; TE = 50) and scapula reveals marrow replacement (M) and soft tissue mass (S) with intermediate signal intensity and apparent intact intervening cortex. However, small areas of linear cortical permeation can be recognized on further evaluation (*open circles*). (*D*) Pictorial illustration reveals intramedullary tumor (M) permeating through the Haversian canals (*arrowheads*) through channels. This pattern of extension allows continuity between the medullary (M) and soft tissue (T) component without focal cortical destruction. (*E, F*) Photographs of coronally sectioned gross specimen (*E*) and whole mount specimen (*F*) (hematoxylin-eosin, original magnification) reveal the cortex (C), medullary canal involvement (M), soft tissue component (S) with continuity seen as focal channels of cortical permeation (*circles*) (original magnification 1X). ([*D–F*] *From* Murphey MD, Senchak LT, Mambalam PK, et al. From the radiologic pathology archives: Ewing sarcoma family of tumors: radiologic-pathologic correlation. Radiographics 2013;33(3):803–31; with permission.)

primary lymphoma of bone shows similar aggressive features as seen radiographically[6,16] (see **Figs. 1–5**). Soft tissue masses associated with the osseous involvement are more commonly seen on CT and MR, as expected (see **Figs. 1–5**). Soft tissue components are seen in 80% of cases by CT and 100% by MR imaging.[1,2,4,7] CT may reveal areas of mineralization, often having an osteoid appearance typically limited to the intraosseous component, in the authors' experience.[17] This appearance represents reactive osteoid and is not typically seen in the extraosseous component of the lesion. The communication between the intraosseous and soft tissue components is often apparent with intervening cortical destruction (see **Figs. 1, 2,** and **5**). However, it is also frequent that the cortex may

appear intact between the 2 components (see **Fig. 3**). At close inspection, small subtle channels of cortical involvement representing extension along vascular channels and the Haversian canals are commonly apparent (see **Fig. 3**). This pattern of extension should always suggest a round blue cell tumor growth pattern. The CT attenuation of the lesion is similar to skeletal muscle with a homogeneous appearance, lacking evidence of necrosis (see **Figs. 1, 2,** and **5**). On MR imaging, the signal intensity is similar to muscle on T1-weighting[18] (see **Figs. 1, 3,** and **4**). There is more variability on T2-weighted MR images with intermediate signal intensity most frequent (60%–70% of cases), likely reflecting the high degree of cellularity in these lesions.[1,2,4,7] High signal intensity on long repetition time (TR)

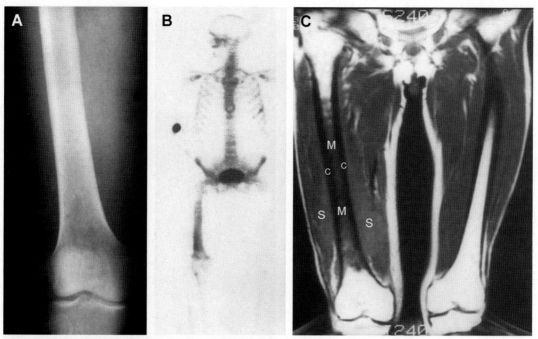

Fig. 4. A 45-year-old woman with lower leg pain. (*A*) Radiograph shows no area of focal bone destruction or sclerosis and appears normal. (*B*) Bone scan reveals diffuse increased radionuclide uptake in the entire femoral shaft. (*C*) Coronal T1-weighted (TR = 500; TE = 25) image demonstrates diffuse marrow replacement (M) and soft tissue mass (S) with normal-appearing intervening cortex (C). Biopsy showed diffuse lymphomatous involvement in both intraosseous and soft tissue components.

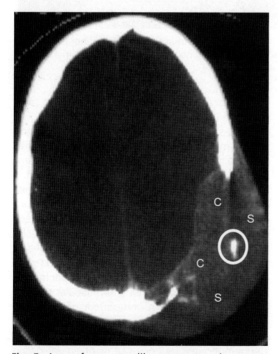

Fig. 5. Area of sequestra-like appearance in osseous lymphoma of the skull in an 80-year-old man. CT shows an aggressive destructive lesion of the calvarium (C) with large soft tissue mass (S). Focal area of sclerosis (*open circle*) represents sequestra-like area.

sequences is seen in 30%–40% of cases.[1,2,4,7] Diffusion-weighted, in and out of phase, and whole body MR imaging have also been used to detect marrow involvement by lymphoma.[18–20] Similar to CT, lesions are often relatively homogeneous, and areas of necrosis or hemorrhage are absent (before therapy). In the authors' experience, prominent surrounding edema in both the soft tissue and the medullary canal is frequent and may simulate an inflammatory process. The authors find this a useful feature because a mass in bone with prominent surrounding edema and lacking pathologic fractures significantly limits the differential diagnosis to osteoid osteoma, osteoblastoma, chondroblastoma, infection, Langerhans cell histiocytosis, and lymphoma. CT reveals an area of sclerosis with a sequestra-like appearance in 33% of cases and is more sensitive compared with radiography in detection of these foci (see **Fig. 5**).

MUSCULOSKELETAL SOFT TISSUE LYMPHOMA

Primary lymphoma of the musculoskeletal soft tissues is also rare. Involvement can occur in the deep soft tissues or cutaneous/subcutaneous tissue. As in other soft tissue masses, MR imaging

A

IT

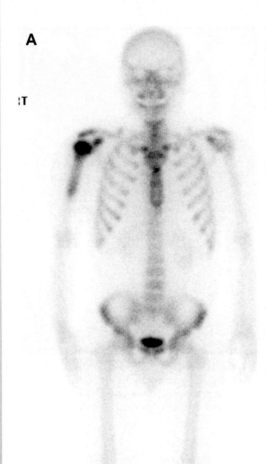

B

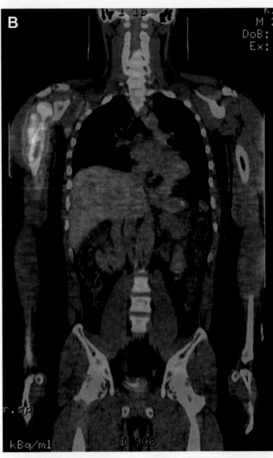

Fig. 6. Bone scintigraphy and FDG-PET images in a 60-year-old man with primary osseous lymphoma of the humerus. (*A*) Coronal bone scan and FDG-PET. (*B*) Images show intense radionuclide uptake in the humeral lesion with associated soft tissue mass (same lesion as depicted in **Fig. 3**B).

is optimal for evaluation owing to its superior contrast resolution.

Lymphoma of the deep soft tissues with muscle involvement has been reported to occur in 1.4% of all musculoskeletal lymphoma.[21–25] The most commonly affected location is the thigh, upper extremities, pelvis, and calf. Radiographs in these patients are typically normal, although soft tissue fullness or mass has been reported.

Nuclear medicine studies in patients with primary soft tissue lymphoma include bone scintigraphy, gallium studies, and FDG-PET.[15,26] Bone scintigraphy usually reveals mild radionuclide uptake in the soft tissue lesion, which is more prominent on blood flow and blood pool images compared with delayed static images. Gallium scintigraphy shows significant radionuclide uptake in soft tissue lymphomatous areas of involvement. FDG-PET studies, similar to other locations, demonstrate intense radionuclide activity in areas of soft tissue lymphoma and has largely supplanted the use of Gallium Scintigraphy.[13,14]

Gallium scintigraphy and FDG-PET have also been used to monitor response to therapy.

Cross-sectional imaging (CT or MR) of deep soft tissue lymphoma shows masses that may be intramuscular or intermuscular (**Fig. 7**). Diffuse intra-articular involvement is also rarely reported.[27] These areas of involvement are often long cones (greater than 15 cm in length) of abnormal lymphomatous masses and are frequently multiple[28] (see **Fig. 7**). The CT attenuation of deep soft tissue lymphomatous involvement is similar to muscle without calcification, and as such, the mass is often difficult to distinguish from normal muscle (see **Fig. 7**). In addition, normal intermuscular fat may be misinterpreted as a component of the lesion suggesting the mistaken diagnosis of liposarcoma. MR imaging more clearly allows distinction of the long lymphomatous cones of involvement owing to the superior contrast resolution of this radiologic modality (see **Fig. 7**). The signal intensity of the lymphomatous tissue is similar to muscle on T1-weighting and intermediate to high signal

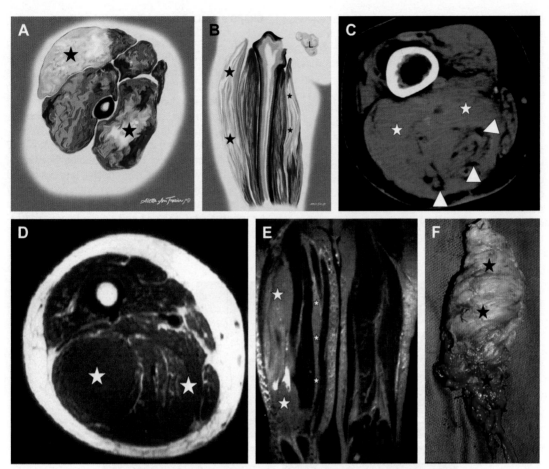

Fig. 7. Deep soft tissue lymphoma of the thigh in a 70-year-old man. (*A, B*) Pictorial representation of the long cones of lymphomatous involvement (*stars*) in axial (*A*) and coronal planes (*B*). Associated lymphadenopathy is also depicted (L). (*C*) Axial CT of the thigh shows soft tissue fullness and mass (*stars*) but intervening compressed intermuscular fat (*arrowheads*) could be mistaken for lesional tissue and diagnosis of liposarcoma. (*D, E*) Axial T1-weighted (*D*, TR = 500; TE = 15) and coronal T2-weighted (*E*, TR = 2000; TE = 100) MR images reveal intermediate signal intensity masses with long cones of involvement (*stars*) on the coronal MR (*E*). The mass shows intermediate signal intensity, and there is edema in the lateral subcutaneous tissue. (*F*) Gross specimen of one of the deep soft tissue masses shows the long cone of lymphomatous tissue (*stars*).

intensity on T2-weighting (see **Fig. 7**). The intermediate signal intensity on water-sensitive MR sequences may be due to the high cellularity of the lymphomatous involvement. Contrast enhancement is mild and diffuse without prominent areas of necrosis or hemorrhage on MR imaging. The lymphomatous cones of involvement may infiltrate into the subcutaneous tissue, and surrounding edema may also be apparent, simulating an inflammatory process. Lee and colleagues[28] reported adjacent abnormal bone marrow signal intensity on MR imaging in 71% of their patients that was much less extensive than the soft tissue involvement. Whether this represents subtle underlying bone involvement or is related to reactive edema is uncertain.

Cutaneous lymphoma can be either T-cell (as in mycosis fungoides) or B-cell disease.[21] Mycosis fungoides accounts for 6% of all non-Hodgkin lymphoma in Europe and is more common in men and blacks. It is an indolent lymphoma often seen initially by dermatologists with eczematous or dermatitis skin lesions. These skin lesions progress to plaquelike areas and ultimately cutaneous masses at which time diagnosis is often established. Extracutaneous involvement (lymphadenopathy and systemic spread) of mycosis fungoides is associated with a marked worsening of prognosis.

Subcutaneous panniculitis-like T-cell lymphoma is a rare lesion first described by Gonzalez and colleagues[29] in 1991. These patients may present clinically with multiple palpable subcutaneous nodules without lymphadenopathy often misinterpreted as inflammatory panniculitis.[21,30] The most common locations are the trunk, extremities, and face.

On cross-sectional imaging (ultrasound, CT, or MR), cutaneous and subcutaneous lymphoma demonstrates nodular foci in the subcutaneous tissue and plaquelike areas of cutaneous thickening and mass formation[21,30,31] (Fig. 8). Ultrasound examination reveals ill-defined hyperechoic areas in the subcutaneous fat with hypervascularity and low resistive index on Doppler evaluation.[30,32–34] On CT and MR, multiple enhancing nodules may be seen replacing the normal subcutaneous fat.[21,30]

BIOPSY AND POSTTHERAPY IMAGING

Biopsy of musculoskeletal lymphoma is vital to establish the diagnosis and distinguish the disease from a primary sarcoma. The importance of this distinction is the difference in treatment between these diseases, with lymphoma being medical chemotherapy in contradistinction to sarcoma, which is primarily surgical. In the authors' experience, biopsy of musculoskeletal lymphoma may be initially interpreted by the pathologist as nondiagnostic owing to the discohesive and collapsed cells.[35] This finding has been emphasized recently by Chang and colleagues[36] with 22% of osseous lymphoma and 17% of soft tissue lymphoma biopsies showing initial nondiagnostic biopsies.

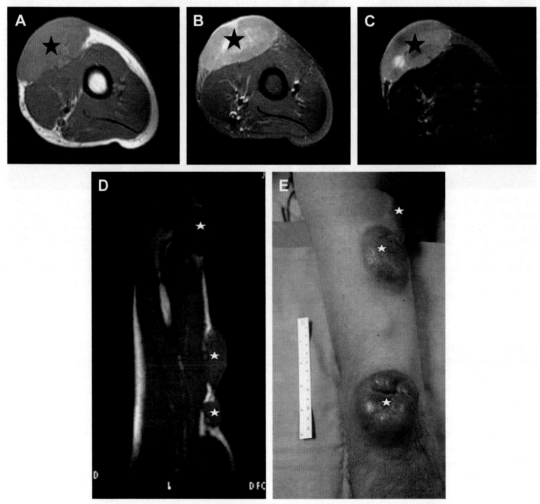

Fig. 8. Cutaneous B-cell lymphoma with multiple cutaneous upper arm masses. (A–C) Axial T1-weighted MR images before and after intravenous contrast (A, B, TR = 500; TE = 20) and T2-weighted (C, TR = 6000; TE = 100) images show a large subcutaneous mass (stars) with intermediate signal intensity and mild diffuse enhancement. (D) Long-axis T1-weighted MR image reveals the multiplicity of subcutaneous masses (stars). (E) These ulcerating subcutaneous masses (stars) are also seen on the clinical photograph.

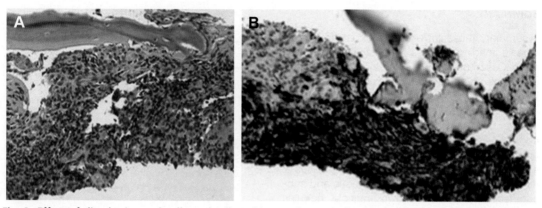

Fig. 9. Effect of discohesive and collapsed cells at biopsy of osseous lymphoma. (*A*) Hematoxylin-eosin stain (original magnification ×100) suggests a nondiagnostic biopsy with discohesive and collapsed cells that are not typical of a round small blue cell tumor, suggesting nondiagnostic biopsy. (*B*) However, because imaging suggested lymphoma, immunohistochemical stains were performed after consultation between the musculoskeletal radiologist and pathologist, revealing intense positive staining for lymphoma (*brown areas*) and obviating repeat biopsy for diagnosis (CD 20 stain, original magnification 100×).

However, in the authors' experience, immunohistochemistry evaluation of these biopsies will still be positive for lymphoma, if performed. In the authors opinion, if the musculoskeletal radiologist emphasizes the possibility of lymphoma as a strong diagnostic consideration from the imaging appearance in collaboration with their pathologic colleagues, the appropriate immunohistochemical evaluation may be performed and alleviate the need for repeat diagnostic biopsy (**Fig. 9**). Further biopsies may still be necessary for lymphoma subtyping.

Posttherapy imaging of primary lymphoma of the musculoskeletal system typically reveals marked reduction in size and extent of the lesion[21,37] (**Fig. 10**). Spontaneous regression of disease is rarely reported.[5] In many cases, residual tumor is not identifiable by CT or MR imaging, representing a dramatic response to therapy[37,38] (see **Fig. 10**). Similarly, FDG-PET imaging reveals a marked reduction of radionuclide activity often returning to normal.[39] The intraosseous component of the lesion may reveal residual or increased sclerosis on radiographs or on CT. Calcification in the residual soft tissue component may also be seen on radiographs and CT with reduced signal intensity on all MR pulse sequences.

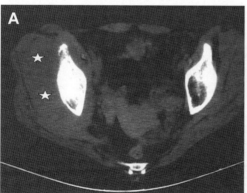
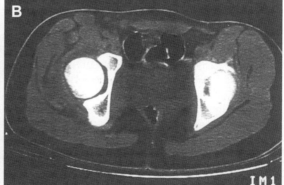

Fig. 10. Treatment effect musculoskeletal lymphoma. (*A*) Axial CT before treatment shows a large lymphomatous mass at the right hip joint (*stars*). (*B*) Axial CT 6 months after initiation of chemotherapy reveals no residual tumor resulting from marked response of the lesion to treatment.

SUMMARY

In summary, musculoskeletal lymphoma frequently reveals imaging features suggestive of the diagnosis. Osseous lymphoma typically shows aggressive bone destruction, which can be associated with a soft tissue mass. Cortical destruction allowing connection between these components may be apparent. However, subtle channellike areas of cortical permeation, typical of small blue cell tumor growth, may also be seen. Lymphoma of the deep soft tissue may demonstrate multiple long cones of neoplasm in the extremities. Cutaneous and subcutaneous lymphoma shows multiple nodules that may develop plaquelike areas of thickening and mass formation. Musculoskeletal lymphoma is one of the few neoplastic processes that may be associated with prominent surrounding edema on MR images. FDG-PET imaging reveals marked increase of radionuclide uptake in areas of musculoskeletal lymphomatous involvement and is useful to assess disease extent. Biopsy of musculoskeletal lymphoma may initially be assessed as nondiagnostic owing to discohesive and collapsed cells. However, immunohistochemistry stains will remain positive, if performed, which may require close collaboration between the musculoskeletal radiologist and pathologist to alleviate the need for repeat diagnostic biopsy. Medical treatment of lymphoma usually results in marked and rapid tumor response, which can be assessed by cross-sectional imaging and FDG-PET. The radiologist is vital in all stages of evaluation of musculoskeletal lymphoma from initial assessment to biopsy and posttreatment to help guide and optimize patient management and outcome.

REFERENCES

1. Mulligan ME, Kransdorf MJ. Sequestra in primary lymphoma of bone: prevalence and radiologic features. AJR Am J Roentgenol 1993;160(6):1245–8.

2. Mulligan ME, McRae GA, Murphey MD. Imaging features of primary lymphoma of bone. AJR Am J Roentgenol 1999;173(6):1691–7.

3. Edeiken-Monroe B, Edeiken J, Kim EE. Radiologic concepts of lymphoma of bone. Radiol Clin North Am 1990;28(4):841–64.

4. Kirsch J, Ilaslan H, Bauer TW, et al. The incidence of imaging findings, and the distribution of skeletal lymphoma in a consecutive patient population seen over 5 years. Skeletal Radiol 2006;35(8):590–4.

5. Mounasamy V, Berns S, Azouz EM, et al. Anaplastic large cell lymphoma presenting as an epiphyseal lytic lesion—a case report with clinico-pathologic correlation. Skeletal Radiol 2006;35(8):619–23.

6. Ruzek KA, Wenger DE. The multiple faces of lymphoma of the musculoskeletal system. Skeletal Radiol 2004;33(1):1–8.

7. Krishnan A, Shirkhoda A, Tehranzadeh J, et al. Primary bone lymphoma: radiographic-MR imaging correlation. Radiographics 2003;23(6):1371–83 [discussion: 1384–7].

8. Heyning F, Kroon HM, Hogendoorn PC, et al. MR imaging characteristics in primary lymphoma of bone with emphasis on non-aggressive appearance. Skeletal Radiol 2007;36(10):937–44.

9. Abdelwahab IF, Hoch B, Hermann G, et al. Primary periosteal lymphoma–rare and unusual. Skeletal Radiol 2007;36(4):335–9.

10. Campbell SE, Filzen TW, Bezzant SM, et al. Primary periosteal lymphoma: an unusual presentation of non-Hodgkin's lymphoma with radiographic, MR imaging, and pathologic correlation. Skeletal Radiol 2003;32(4):231–5.

11. Goudarzi B, Jacene HA, Wahl RL. Measuring the "unmeasurable": assessment of bone marrow response to therapy using FDG-PET in patients with lymphoma. Acad Radiol 2010;17(9):1175–85.

12. Otero HJ, Jagannathan JP, Prevedello LM, et al. CT and PET/CT findings of T-cell lymphoma. AJR Am J Roentgenol 2009;193(2):349–58.

13. Metser U, Goor O, Lerman H, et al. PET-CT of extranodal lymphoma. AJR Am J Roentgenol 2004;182(6):1579–86.

14. Kazama T, Faria SC, Varavithya V, et al. FDG PET in the evaluation of treatment for lymphoma: clinical usefulness and pitfalls. Radiographics 2005;25(1):191–207.

15. Orzel JA, Sawaf NW, Richardson ML. Lymphoma of the skeleton: scintigraphic evaluation. AJR Am J Roentgenol 1988;150(5):1095–9.

16. Malloy PC, Fishman EK, Magid D. Lymphoma of bone, muscle, and skin: CT findings. AJR Am J Roentgenol 1992;159(4):805–9.

17. Apter S, Avigdor A, Gayer G, et al. Calcification in lymphoma occurring before therapy: CT features and clinical correlation. AJR Am J Roentgenol 2002;178(4):935–8.

18. Yasumoto M, Nonomura Y, Yoshimura R, et al. MR detection of iliac bone marrow involvement by malignant lymphoma with various MR sequences including diffusion-weighted echo-planar imaging. Skeletal Radiol 2002;31(5):263–9.

19. Shields AF, Porter BA, Churchley S, et al. The detection of bone marrow involvement by lymphoma using magnetic resonance imaging. J Clin Oncol 1987;5(2):225–30.

20. Stiglbauer R, Augustin I, Kramer J, et al. MRI in the diagnosis of primary lymphoma of bone: correlation with histopathology. J Comput Assist Tomogr 1992;16(2):248–53.

21. Lee HJ, Im JG, Goo JM, et al. Peripheral T-cell lymphoma: spectrum of imaging findings with clinical and pathologic features. Radiographics 2003; 23(1):7–26.
22. ter Braak BP, Guit GL, Bloem JL. Case 111: soft-tissue lymphoma. Radiology 2007;243(1): 293–6.
23. Grunshaw ND, Chalmers AG. Skeletal muscle lymphoma. Clin Radiol 1992;45(6):399–400.
24. Metzler JP, Fleckenstein JL, Vuitch F, et al. Skeletal muscle lymphoma: MRI evaluation. Magn Reson Imaging 1992;10(3):491–4.
25. Eustace S, Winalski CS, McGowen A, et al. Skeletal muscle lymphoma: observations at MR imaging. Skeletal Radiol 1996;25(5):425–30.
26. Bar-Shalom R, Israel O, Epelbaum R, et al. Gallium-67 scintigraphy in lymphoma with bone involvement. J Nucl Med 1995;36:446–50.
27. Donovan A, Schweitzer ME, Garcia RA, et al. Chronic lymphocytic leukemia/small lymphocytic lymphoma presenting as septic arthritis of the shoulder. Skeletal Radiol 2008;37(11):1035–9.
28. Lee VS, Martinez S, Coleman RE. Primary muscle lymphoma: clinical and imaging findings. Radiology 1997;203(1):237–44.
29. Gonzalez CL, Medeiros LJ, Braziel RM, et al. T-cell lymphoma involving subcutaneous tissue. A clinicopathologic entity commonly associated with hemophagocytic syndrome. Am J Surg Pathol 1991; 15(1):17–27.
30. Kang BS, Choi SH, Cha HJ, et al. Subcutaneous panniculitis-like T-cell lymphoma: US and CT findings in three patients. Skeletal Radiol 2007;36(1): S67–71.
31. Nessi R, Betti R, Bencini PL, et al. Ultrasonography of nodular and infiltrative lesions of the skin and subcutaneous tissues. J Clin Ultrasound 1990;18(2): 103–9.
32. Chiou HJ, Chou YH, Chiou SY, et al. High-resolution ultrasonography of primary peripheral soft tissue lymphoma. J Ultrasound Med 2005;24(1): 77–86.
33. Giovagnorio F. Sonography of cutaneous non-Hodgkin's lymphomas. Clin Radiol 1997;52(4): 301–3.
34. Fujii Y, Shinozaki T, Koibuchi H, et al. Primary peripheral T-cell lymphoma in subcutaneous tissue: sonographic findings. J Clin Ultrasound 2004;32(7): 361–4.
35. Peng SL, Cheng CN, Chang KC. Burkitt lymphoma with Azzopardi phenomenon. Arch Pathol Lab Med 2007;131(5):682–3.
36. Chang CY, Huang AJ, Bredella MA, et al. Percutaneous CT-guided needle biopsies of musculoskeletal tumors: a 5-year analysis of non-diagnostic biopsies. Skeletal Radiol 2015; 44(12):1795–803.
37. Mengiardi B, Honegger H, Hodler J, et al. Primary lymphoma of bone: MRI and CT characteristics during and after successful treatment. AJR Am J Roentgenol 2005;184(1):185–92.
38. Johnson SA, Kumar A, Matasar MJ, et al. Imaging for staging and response assessment in lymphoma. Radiology 2015;276(2):323–38.
39. Okada J, Yoshikawa K, Imazeki K, et al. The use of FDG-PET in the detection and management of malignant lymphoma: correlation of uptake with prognosis. J Nucl Med 1991;32(4):686–91.

Index

Note: Page numbers of article titles are in **boldface** type.

Radiol Clin N Am 54 (2016) 797–800
http://dx.doi.org/10.1016/S0033-8389(16)30050-1
0033-8389/16/$ – see front matter

Moving?

Make sure your subscription moves with you!

To notify us of your new address, find your **Clinics Account Number** (located on your mailing label above your name), and contact customer service at:

Email: journalscustomerservice-usa@elsevier.com

800-654-2452 (subscribers in the U.S. & Canada)
314-447-8871 (subscribers outside of the U.S. & Canada)

Fax number: 314-447-8029

Elsevier Health Sciences Division
Subscription Customer Service
3251 Riverport Lane
Maryland Heights, MO 63043

*To ensure uninterrupted delivery of your subscription, please notify us at least 4 weeks in advance of move.